DON'T GET SICK IN AMERICA

To Lisbeth Bamberger Schorr,
whose book this also is in so many ways.

DON'T GET SICK IN AMERICA
By DANIEL SCHORR

Aurora Publishers Incorporated
NASHVILLE AND LONDON

COPYRIGHT © 1970 BY
COLUMBIA BROADCASTING SYSTEM
NEW YORK CITY AND
AURORA PUBLISHERS INCORPORATED
NASHVILLE, TENNESSEE 37219
LIBRARY OF CONGRESS CATALOG CARD NUMBER: 70-129023
STANDARD BOOK NUMBER: 87695-103-5
MANUFACTURED IN THE UNITED STATES OF AMERICA

CONTENTS

PREFACE –6

INTRODUCTION By Senator Edward M. Kennedy –7

I. FROM INVESTIGATION TO CONTROVERSY –17

II. CASE HISTORIES IN FAILURE –23

III. THE "CORNER GROCERY" HOSPITAL –45

IV. THE "PUSHCART PEDDLER" DOCTOR –77

V. HEALTH INSURANCE: THE SHRINKING SECURITY BLANKET –87

VI. THE TRAUMA OF MEDICARE AND MEDICAID –101

VII. "KEEP WELL!": THE DRIVE FOR HEALTH MAINTENANCE –113

VIII. BRINGING THE POOR INTO THE HEALTH SYSTEM –131

IX. HOW THEY DO IT OVER THERE –147

X. THE DRIVE FOR NATIONAL HEALTH INSURANCE –163

APPENDIX ONE –187

APPENDIX TWO –204

APPENDIX THREE –209

PREFACE

When President Nixon speaks of a "massive crisis" in the delivery of health care and *Fortune* magazine sees American medicine standing "on the brink of chaos," there is clearly a subject for investigation. This investigation, leading to two-hour-long CBS Reports' documentaries on successive nights, was a major project of CBS News in 1970, and it produced a major controversy. This book is a more complete report of that inquiry.

CBS Reports' "Health in America" was the result of a team effort and months of research. On the first broadcast, George Herman was the reporter, Irv Drasnin the producer, and Joseph Zigman and Alvin H. Goldstein the associate producers. On the second broadcast Gene DePoris was the producer, David Lowe the associate producer, and I was the reporter. Burton Benjamin, as executive producer of both broadcasts, provided helpful insights.

In this book I have drawn on the work of all my colleagues and of the research assistants who backed us up, all of which I gratefully acknowledge. But this book reflects my organization of material, analysis, and conclusions, and for them I accept responsibility.

This is frankly a view of the health industry as perceived by the consumer rather than the supplier. It is the patient more than the doctor who is in trouble. It is he, ultimately, who will require a long-overdue change in America's health-care system.

—Daniel Schorr

INTRODUCTION
BY SENATOR EDWARD M. KENNEDY

In the United States of 1970, health care is the fastest growing failing business—a $63 billion industry that fails to meet the urgent demands of our people. Today, more than ever before, we are spending more on health care and enjoying it less. By 1975, we are told, we may be spending $100 billion a year on health and be worse off than we are now in terms of the quality and responsiveness of our health-care system.

In spite of the fact that our vaunted research and technology are unequalled by any other nation in the history of the world, America is an also-ran in the delivery of health care to people. In areas like infant mortality, maternal mortality, life expectancy, and death rate for middle-aged citizens, America lags far behind almost every nation in Western Europe. At the same time, the billions of dollars we pour into our inadequate health system are more than is spent by any other nation in the world, either in absolute terms or as a percent of Gross National Product.

As this extraordinary volume by Daniel Schorr makes clear, we cannot go on subsidizing our present failures, patching the existing system beyond any hope of repair. We must begin the long journey toward real reform, toward revolutionizing the system, toward comprehensive change in the organization, delivery, and financing of health care in America.

I believe that we have already witnessed the first skirmishes in a "patients' revolt." The revolt is gaining in momentum. Indeed, it is beginning to rival, in intensity, the taxpayers' revolt of 1969, which culminated in the most far-reaching tax reform legislation in our history.

If we are to be equal to the challenge that exists, we must be prepared to take major steps. Hippocrates put it well two thousand years ago when he said that where the illness is extreme, extreme treatment may be necessary. As a legislator concerned with charting the proper Federal role, I am convinced that there are a number of major steps we must take if we are to improve the quality of health care for our citizens.

We need a new approach to the politics of health. Our single greatest deficiency in the area of health is our failure to develop a national health constituency, committed to a progressive and enlightened health policy. The issue is far more serious than the simple question of braking the momentum of the status quo. Today all too often, whether the area is medicine, or education, or pollution, the vested interests are strongly ranged against innovation, and there is no champion capable of marshaling the diffuse advocates for progress and reform. When a better teaching organization threatens the bureaucratic status quo in education, we know there will be organized advocacy by parents and children. When a new and more efficient development is offered that threatens the status quo in health—whether in the organization, financing, or delivery of health care—we know there will be opposition from organized medicine, but there is seldom organized advocacy by health consumers.

A thorough consideration of the relative merits of alternative proposals is made difficult, if not impossible, by the presence of powerful spokesmen for the old and the absence of effective spokesmen for the new. If we are to succeed in making basic changes in our health-care system, we can do so only by creating the sort of progressive national health constituency that can make itself heard in the halls of Congress and the councils of organized medicine.

We need new institutions at all levels—Federal, state, local, public, and private. Leaders of the health profession must make an even greater effort to lend their expert knowledge and technology to transform American medicine out of its "cottage industry" stereotype, and replace it with a structure capable of meeting the contemporary needs of our people.

The Federal Government must play a far more active and coherent role in the formulation, coordination, and implementation of the health policy. Perhaps the most serious fault in the present situation is the fragmentation and decentralization of the Federal role in health. The $18 billion in Federal outlays for health for 1970 are divided among twenty-four

INTRODUCTION

separate departments and agencies. By far the largest amount—$13 billion—is expended by the Department of Health, Education, and Welfare (HEW), but significant amounts are also expended by the Department of Defense—$2 billion—and the Veterans Administration—$1.7 billion.

Unbelievable as it may seem, the vast array of Federal health programs operate in a policy vacuum. As a nation we have never attempted to formulate a national health policy. We do not even have the mechanism to coordinate health activities in HEW, let alone in all the various Federal health programs that exist in other departments and agencies. The nation's top health officer—the assistant secretary for Health and Scientific Affairs in HEW—has direct authority and control over only sixteen percent of total Federal health spending and over only twenty-two percent of total HEW health spending. Medicare and Medicaid, and a number of other health programs in HEW, are completely outside his jurisdiction.

We cannot afford this bewildering maze of overlapping and conflicting Federal health programs. We must develop a comprehensive and carefully coordinated national health policy, with an administrative structure capable of setting health goals and priorities for the nation. In the spring of 1968, I introduced legislation in Congress to create a National Council of Health Advisers, to be established in the executive office of the President, with responsibility for setting health policies and making recommendations for the attainment of health goals, including the evaluation, coordination, and consolidation of all Federal health programs and activities. The council would be modeled along the lines of the Council of Economic Advisers, which has consistently played a superlative and highly professional role in planning and coordinating the nation's economic policy. I am hopeful now that this council will come into being.

We must give special attention to the health of our urban and rural poor. For too many of the poor, the only "doctor" they know is the cold and impersonal emergency ward of the municipal or county hospital. For too many of our citizens, the family physician has disappeared, to be replaced by the endless lines and depressing waiting rooms of hospitals built at the turn of the century. Yet, there are few physicians today who were not trained on the wards and charity patients of our teaching hospitals. Too often, as Professor Alonzo Yerby has eloquently stated, our poor have had to barter their bodies and their dignity in return for medical treatment.

Nowhere are the inequalities of our society more obvious than in the sickness of our poor. We know that our affluent few can buy the world's best medical care. But all too often it is care provided in modern medical towers looking out on urban landscapes, condemning thousands of citizens to a lifetime of disease, under some of the worst medical care anywhere in the world.

In the United States today—the wealthiest nation in the history of man—millions of our citizens are sick. And they are sick because they are poor. Their sickness is the shame of America. Of all the faces of poverty, the sickness of the poor is the ugliest. Of all the effects of poverty, it is the sickness of the poor that we could attack most easily—had we the will.

The difference in health care between the rich and the poor is measured by the stunted bodies, shortened lives, and physical handicaps of those who live in poverty. The President's Riot Commission found that the nation is moving toward two societies—one black, one white—separate and unequal. That conclusion was starkly documented by the commission in the existing pattern of unequal health care that is widening the gulf that divides our society.

At the very least, we ought to create a national health corps as an alternative to the draft for doctors, along the lines of the "Project USA" program recently recommended by the American Medical Association. Today doctors are exempt from the draft if they serve two years in the National Institutes of Health or in other branches of the public health service. The same exemption should apply to doctors volunteering for medical service in urban or rural poverty areas. Only in this way will we be able to meet the critical need for health manpower in depressed areas. Once young physicians are exposed to the problems of health care for the poor, a significant number will be encouraged to remain and dedicate their careers to this service.

In addition, we ought to make a substantial new effort to expand the neighborhood health-center program. At the present time, fewer than a dozen medical societies in the nation have become actively involved in neighborhood health centers. Yet, in recent months, prominent leaders of the American Medical Association have called for a greater role for neighborhood health centers as a means of extending health care to the poor. A few imaginative pilot projects reaching in this direction have recently been funded by the Office of Economic Opportunity, including a program to reorganize the out-patient department at Boston City Hospital as a nucleus for community health care, but our overall effort has been inadequate. Tragically, at a time when even organized medicine is moving forward, we have been unwilling to allocate the resources that are so urgently needed for this program.

We must restore the severe budget cuts that have been made in Federal health programs by the Administration. At this time of medical crisis, Federal assistance to health programs is being drastically curtailed, especially in the crucial areas of research, services, and manpower.

The high price we are paying for the war in Viet Nam abroad and the fight against inflation at home has special relevance to the area of health. The impact of the budget cuts will be felt in medical schools, universities, and research centers throughout the nation. The cost of the reductions is far more than the dollars and cents involved. It will be measured in terms of research cut short, medical advances unrealized, new fields unexplored, devastating diseases uncured, and, worst of all, it will be measured by the loss of promising young men and women from careers in the life sciences.

Finally, we must begin to move now to establish a comprehensive national health insurance program, capable of bringing the same amount of high-quality health care to every man, woman, and child in the United States.

National health insurance is an idea whose time has been long in coming. Today, the United States is the only major industrial nation in the world that does not have a national health service or a program of national health insurance. The first comprehensive compulsory national health insurance was enacted in Prussia in 1854. Throughout the twentieth century, proposals have been periodically raised for an American program but never, until recently, with great chance of success.

National health insurance was a major proposal of Theodore Roosevelt during his campaign for the Presidency in 1912. Shortly before World War I a similar proposal managed to gain the support of the American Medical Association, whose orientation then was far different than it is today. During the debate on social security in the thirties, the issue was again raised but without success.

Today the prospect is better. In large part, it is better because of the popularity of Medicare and the fact that many other great national health programs have been successfully launched. The need for national health insurance has become more compelling, and its absence is more conspicuous. In part, the prospect is good because the popular demand for change in our existing health system is consolidating urgent and widespread new support for a national health insurance program as a way out of the present crisis.

For more than two years, I have been privileged to serve as a member of the Committee for National Health Insurance, founded by Walter Reuther, whose goal has been to mobilize broad public support for a national health insurance program in the United States.

The tragedy of Walter Reuther's sudden death is compounded by the fact that his life was cut short at its prime, when he was on the threshold of achieving one of his greatest social goals, a national health insurance program to bring adequate health care to every American. Just as the great scientist, Lord Rutherford, when asked how he always happened to be riding the crest of the wave of modern physics, is said to have replied, "I made the wave, didn't I?" so Walter Reuther helped to make the wave of the health revolution that is cresting in America. Now that the Reuther proposal for national health insurance has been introduced in Congress, I believe it is fair to say that it is the single most important, imaginative, and farsighted legislation introduced in the present Congress, whether in health or any other area. In the years to come, when Congress finally responds to the demand of the American people for better health, the legislation we enact for national health insurance will be a living memorial to Walter Reuther.

A great deal of solid groundwork has already been laid toward establishing a national health insurance program. The time has come to transfer the debate from the halls of the universities and the offices of professors to the public arena—to the hearing rooms of Congress and to the offices of the elected representatives.

This is an issue we can and must take to the people. We can achieve our goal only through the mobilization of millions of decent Americans, concerned with the high cost and inadequate organization and delivery of health care in the nation.

In 1969, in Congress, as I have said, we witnessed the culmination of what has been one of the most powerful nationwide legislative reform movements since I joined the Senate—the taxpayers' revolution. We need the same sort of national effort for health—we need a national health revolution, a revolution by the consumers of health care that will stimulate action by Congress and produce a more equitable health system.

In light of the substantial groundwork already laid, I believe there are four principles we should pursue in preparing an effective program for national health insurance:

1. Most important, our guiding principle should be that the amount and quality of medical care an individual receives is not a function of his income. There should be no difference between health care for the suburbs and health care for the ghetto, between health care for the rich and health care for the poor.

2. The program should be as broad and as

comprehensive as possible, with the maximum free choice available to each health consumer in selecting the care he receives.

3. The costs of the program should be borne on a progressive basis, related to the income level of those who participate in the program.

4. The program cannot be simply an insurance program. It must also contain strong incentives to improve the existing system for organization and delivery of health care in the United States.

We know from recent experience that changes in the organization and delivery system will come only by an excruciating national effort. Throughout our society today, there is perhaps no institution more resistant to change than the organized medical profession. Indeed, because the crisis is so serious in the organization and delivery of health care, there are many who argue that we must make improvements in the organization and delivery system before we can safely embark on changing the financing system through national health insurance.

I believe the opposite is true. We must use the financing mechanism to create strong new incentives for reorganization and delivery of health care. Thomas Paine declared at the founding of our American republic, echoing the words of the ancient Greeks, "Give us a lever and we shall move the world." I say, give us the lever of national health insurance, and together we shall move the medical world and achieve the reforms that are so desperately needed.

The fact that the time has come for national health insurance makes it all the more urgent to pour new resources into remaking our present system. The organization and delivery of health care is so obviously inadequate to meet our current health crisis that only the catalyst of national health insurance will be able to produce the sort of basic revolution that is needed if we are to escape the twin evils of a national health disaster or the federalization of health care in the seventies. To those who say that national health insurance won't work unless we *first* have an enormous increase in health manpower and health facilities and a revolution in the delivery of health care, I reply that *until* we begin moving toward national health insurance, neither Congress nor the medical profession will ever take the basic steps that are essential to reorganize the system. Without national health insurance to galvanize us into action, I fear that we will simply continue to patch the present system beyond any reasonable hope of survival.

The need for comprehensive national health insurance and concomitant changes in the organization and delivery of health care in the United States is the single most important issue of health policy today. If we are to reach our goal of bringing adequate health care to all our citizens, we must have full and generous cooperation between Congress, the administration, and the health profession. We already possess the knowledge and the technology to achieve our goal. This book by Daniel Schorr gives us an eloquent documentation of the need. All we require is the will. The challenge is enormous, but I am confident that we are equal to the task.

CHAPTER I
FROM INVESTIGATION TO CONTROVERSY

American medicine has written many glorious pages. You will not find those pages in this book. Not because we lack admiration for the miracles wrought by American medicine, but because our subject is the difficulty that Americans find in gaining access to these miracles within their means. We have explored not what is right, but what is wrong with American health care—how it is delivered, how it is organized, how it is paid.

We wanted to know why the world's wealthiest nation is far from being the healthiest; why the cost keeps zooming more than twice as fast as other consumer costs, taking a bigger and bigger bite out of our Gross National Product (from 4.5 to 6.8 percent in twenty years); why, for more than $63 billion a year, the American public is not getting anything like adequate health care; and why in America a baby's chance of surviving its first month is worse than in fourteen other countries, its mother's chance of surviving delivery worse than in seventeen other countries. American health services are certainly not meeting the needs of the poor and, as some shocked people are discovering, are no longer meeting the needs of the middle-class.

The new grumblers are the middle-income Americans, complaining, not only about long delays in the doctor's office or the doctor who won't make house calls, but also about the $100-a-day hospital bed and the rising health insurance premiums, which may still not cover some of the whopping bills. While minority problems tend to be overlooked, health care is turning into a majority problem.

Sadly, the average American is inclined to express his resentment at his immediate point of contact with the health system—the doctor and the hospital. It is a fact that never has there been such a chasm of frustration between the American and his healers. The image of the selfless doctor has been gradually changing, in the American mind, to that of a callous, overpaid, high-living, Cadillac-riding businessman. Dr. Kildare has dissolved into Dr. Scrooge, and the hospital has changed shape, in popular fantasy, from a misty haven of healing to a nightmarish ever-jingling cash-register.

FROM INVESTIGATION TO CONTROVERSY

This is unfortunate because the problem goes far beyond the usually conscientious practitioner and the overworked hospital administrator, themselves as much victims as beneficiaries of a creaky health system that is no longer able to meet the rising needs and the rising expectations of Americans. Some of the practitioners and administrators defend the status quo, and some do not. Among those who do not there is widespread disagreement about solutions. In general, as an organized body they tend to resist change and are hostile to outside intervention into what they consider their affairs.

But the organization of health care has become too grave a problem to be left to doctors, just as war has become too important to be managed by soldiers. The doctors who can so skillfully treat disease have demonstrated their lack of ability, if not will, to cure the galloping inflation and fragmentation afflicting their own collective body. Or, as a Federal task force more tactfully put it, "The day is past when doctors and hospital administrators and trustees and their associates may rely only on their judgments of how they can best distribute all the skills and resources at their disposal to what they see as the greatest advantage for the people they think they should be serving."

For diagnosis, prognosis, and prescription, we turned, in the course of our investigation, to many non-practitioners—to some patients and would-be patients, to some administrators concerned with health—in and out of Government. We found it particularly fruitful to turn to that little band of academic experts called the medical economists, the systems analysts of the health industry. We turned also to the American Medical Association, but the critical thrust of our inquiry must have been too evident, for we became aware that the medical establishment was coming to regard us as an adversary.

The two hours of CBS Reports on "Health in America" produced a massive spasm of telephone calls, telegrams, and letters that made it clear we had touched a raw nerve. Or, more precisely, two nerves—one in the health industry and one in the American public.

A surgeon in Richardson, Texas, said, "I do not believe

that I have ever seen a more biased and one-sided view of health care and the health profession in all of my life."

But a lady in Arcata, California, told how she and her husband had worked long hours trying to pay their medical bills and said, "Yes, its true, if you live in America and you're sick, you're really in trouble. . . . I can put you in contact with other people who are as dissatisfied as I am, but don't know what to do about it."

The wife of a pediatrician in Shreveport, Louisiana, wrote, "My husband worked from 8 A.M. until 6 P.M., left home again at 9 P.M. It is 11 P.M. now, and I don't know yet when he will be home again. Is it wrong that I expect society to judge my husband as a kind and just person until he proves himself otherwise?"

But a lady in Lakeland, Florida, wrote, "This letter is to thank you for finally exposing the inhuman way most of the people in this country are treated by the doctors of this country."

A doctor in Bloomington, Indiana, telegraphed, ". . . your presentation was hogwash. . . . American medicine has always taken care of the American public and always will, perhaps not in the red carpet manner, but nevertheless has taken care of them."

But a married couple in Chicago, Illinois, wrote, "Please accept our humble gratitude. . . . What can we as private citizens do? We need a national health program and we plead for instructions so our efforts can be constructive."

The wife of a physician in industrial medicine in Dallas, Texas, complained, "He has not had a vacation in over two years, and probably won't be able to go on one in the near future. . . . We use the telephone to carry on the business of our marriage. Answer me this, gentlemen, what more do you expect from my husband?"

But a lady in Oklahoma City, Oklahoma, wrote, "Having had a great deal of chronic illness in our family of five, we have had much first-hand experience with doctors. . . . I am a very conservative Republican, but would vote for socialized medicine today if given the opportunity."

Last but not least, the American Medical Association called the broadcasts "slanted, totally unbalanced, and a disservice to medicine," and proposed, at its 1970 convention in Chicago, to mount a five-year, $10 million campaign on television to improve the image of organized medicine.

But, Dr. James Cavanaugh, Deputy Assistant Secretary for Health in HEW, told the American Assembly in Harriman, New York, "Despite overwhelming evidence that many millions of people are not receiving adequate health services, despite flagrant maldistribution of health resources, despite these clear signs of impending collapse of the health-care system, we still find among us those who argue that everything is all right. They talk as though the health-care system needed only to be left alone to lick its wounds. Well, wound-licking won't be good enough. The wounds are too deep, too badly infected. Unless they get prompt attention, the patient, the pluralistic health-care system as we know it in this country, may not—in all probability *will not*—pull through."

It was perhaps inevitable that two hours of prime-time television, focussing on the shortcomings of health care in America and bluntly bringing to the foreground some highly sensitive proposals for improvement, would stir a controversy. This book is a further elaboration on the same themes, and it may stir further controversy.

CHAPTER II
CASE HISTORIES IN FAILURE

DON'T GET SICK IN AMERICA

Millions of Americans cannot get health care when they need it—in some cases because they cannot pay for the services, in some cases because the services are simply not there. For illustrations of medical insecurity in a country of medical breakthroughs, highly trained professionals, and a network of splendid hospitals, we crossed the continent. One case took us across the ocean to talk to a man priced not only out of the American health market but out of America. His sorrowful judgment suggested the title of this book. So, let us start with the story of the man exiled from the country by the high price of staying alive.

Nymegen, Holland: "Don't Get Sick in America!"

In 1957, Johan van der Sande, thirty-three, an accountant from Nymegen, the Netherlands, brought his wife, Yvette, to find a new life in the United States. They settled down in Monrovia, California, where her brother lived. Life was rough at first and the homesick Van der Sande considered returning to Holland. But his brother wrote from Nymegen reminding him that he would have to live the rest of his life oppressed by the feeling of not having been able to make it in America. So, he determined to make it. He applied himself to learning English, Americanized his name to "John," finally found a good job, and adopted two children. By 1965, Van der Sande felt like "a real Californian," with a $1,000-a-month job as a certified public accountant, a family, and a heavily mortgaged home in nearby Arcadia.

Then, having cleared all the known obstacles, Van der Sande suddenly confronted the health hurdle. In 1966, he started suffering from high blood pressure. Sometimes his mind would go blank, and he found he could not function adequately. Several times he changed jobs while keeping himself going with four "blood-pressure pills" and four tranquilizers a day.

In 1969, his problem was diagnosed as a kidney ailment, and he entered Mt. Sinai Medical Center in Los Angeles. There he received dialysis treatment—was attached to an artificial kidney machine—at a cost of $200 to $300 per treatment. Out of work and unable to meet mortgage payments, he proposed to sell his house. His doctor forbade this, saying it was important to his recovery that he return to familiar surroundings.

By the time he left the hospital, his bills added up to a staggering $22,000. The first $20,000 of his bill was covered by his Blue Cross policy. But from then on the home dialysis unit he needed to stay alive, though cheaper than hospital treatment in the long run, meant a first-year investment of $25,000 and $5,000 a year.

A group of friends formed a "Van der Sande Kidney Fund" to support his treatment, raising money by such ventures as a fashion show. But it is difficult to sustain such generosity over a long period. Contributions began to taper off, and Van der Sande faced the problem of how to stay alive.

From his family in Holland came a suggestion—since he had neglected to adopt American citizenship, he still had health-care rights in the old country. Come home! California friends felt that this meant defeat for them but agreed that there seemed no other way. "In America," says Van der Sande, "even if I could get help, I would have to be dependent on charity. I would have to hold out my hand and say, 'Will you help me please?'"

So, in 1969, Van der Sande returned to Holland. There, under the National Health Insurance plan, for a premium of $24 a month, he receives full coverage of hospital, doctors', and drug bills—and an artificial kidney developed in the United States. CBS News Correspondent Morley Safer went to Nymegen to see how Van der Sande, once again Johan instead of John, is faring—and whether he misses America. The man who almost made it in America lives now in a modest row house and says:

"I miss the freedom, the open spaces, and the sunshine. I didn't like to leave. I feel my roots are still in California. People here were amazed at what friends did for me in California. But in Holland that would not be necessary. In Holland you have a right. The taxpayers pay into a fund, and everybody has a right to be taken care of. America has

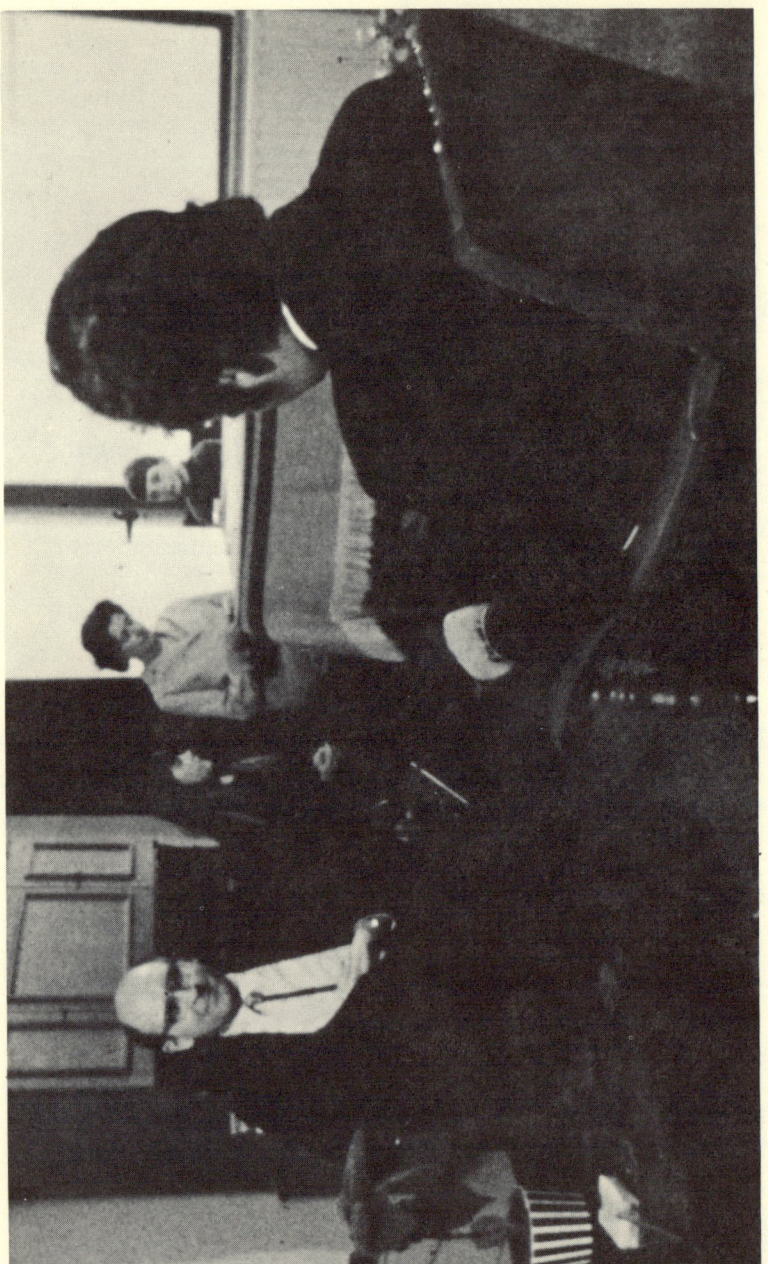

"My roots are still in California."

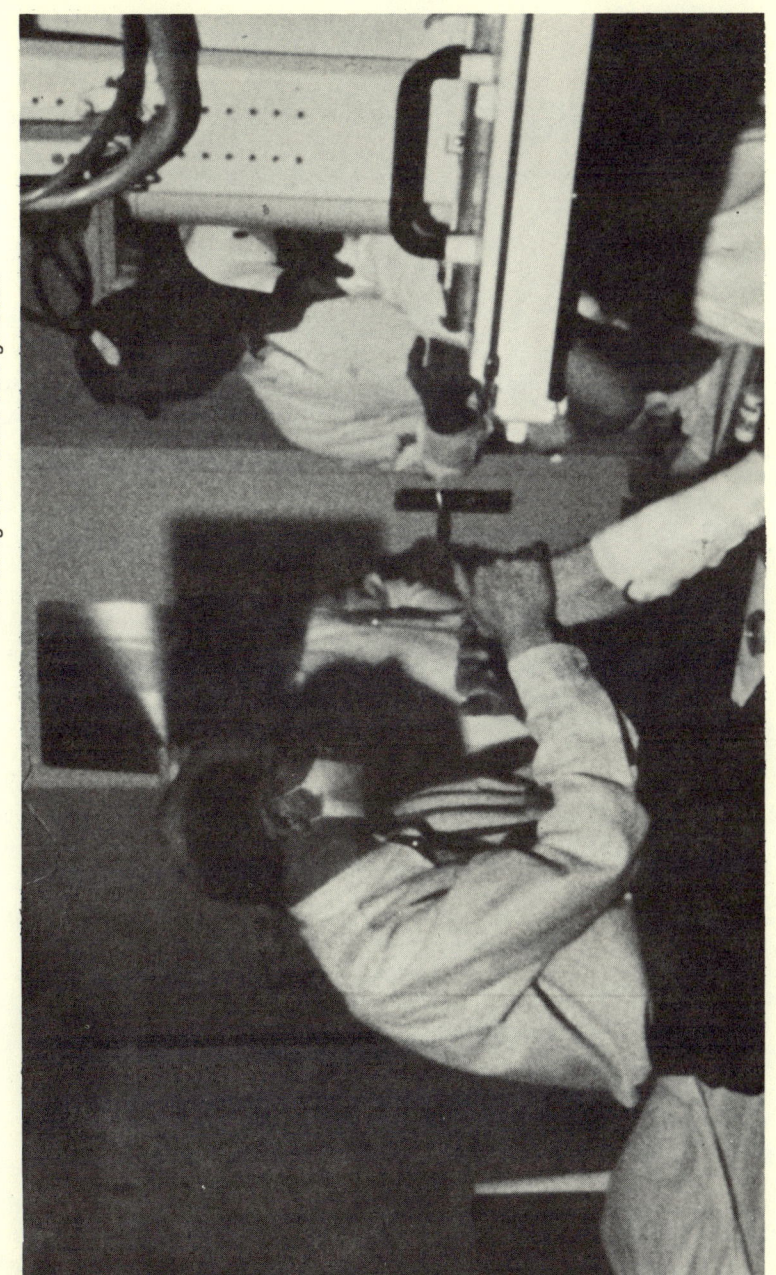

"... being sick I don't dare go back."

a system where, at some point, you may be left alone unless private citizens come together to help you. And then you have to say, 'Thank you again,' and that is not pleasant.

"If I were a healthy person, I would go back to America tomorrow. But, being sick, I don't dare to go back to America. I feel that America is a good place to live if you're healthy. But don't get sick in America!"

* * *

Wolcott, Indiana: Is There a Doctor in the Town?
Bob Foster, the local funeral director, is an important man in life as well as death. His hearse has done double duty as an ambulance to take the stricken to the doctor, sometimes as far as thirty miles away. Wolcott, a comfortable town of 8,000, living off the land, can easily afford a doctor, but like 5,000 small communities in the hustings, it has trouble getting one. Today, with 8,000 doctors a year coming out of medical school, few choose to treat patients, and most of these few prefer to live in the cities or in the suburbs. So, for two years, Wolcott had no doctor.

Correspondent George Herman heard the consequences of this in conversations in Nordyke's Drug Store, the chief local center for health care.

A woman said, "We had a five-year-old boy that got sick in the middle of the night. And then, I think, that's when you really notice most that you can't get any help. I couldn't get a doctor to come to the house, so we just had to take him to the hospital in Lafayette."

A man said, "When I don't feel well, I come to Doc Nordyke, and I say, 'Doc, you gotta fix me up.' And he gives me something."

Pharmacist Bob Nordyke said, "They used to go to the doctor with their ailments. Now they come in and say, 'What do you have for the twenty-four hour flu?' and that sort of thing. I think that my major job is to tell them that I've got something for them that will help, or say, 'Your problem

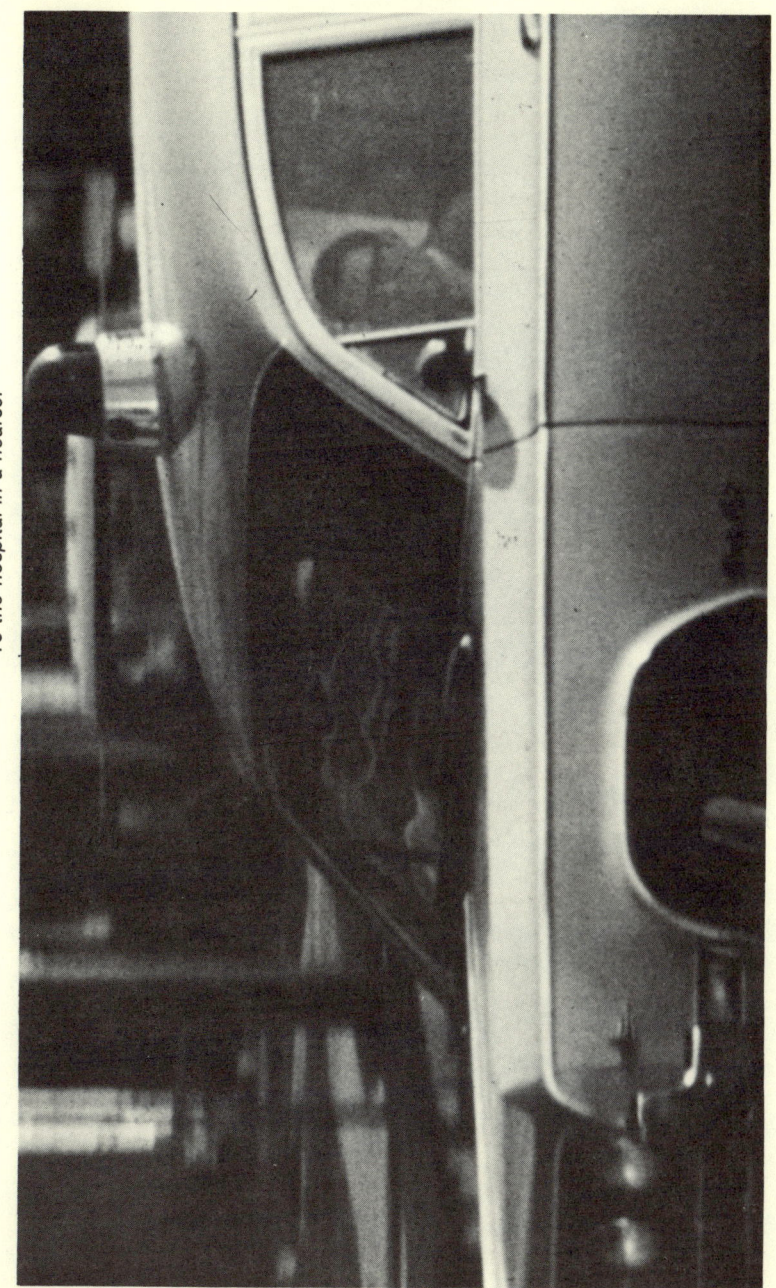

To the hospital in a hearse.

is a little too serious, and you'd better get in touch with the doctor.'"

For emergencies there is Bob Foster. Then it's a thirty-mile ride in the hearse-ambulance to the hospital in Lafayette.

Some residents told their problems in the local tavern.

"I had a man working for me, and he had a coronary heart attack at seven o'clock in the morning. It was winter and pitch dark. And before anything could be done for him, he was dead. I feel that if there had been a doctor available, that man would have been alive today. He was thirty-nine years old. . . . "

"I went to a doctor in Rensselaer. The man's got more than he can take care of. You go to Remington, and they turn you down. You just can't get any help. In all those places you're lucky if you can get in to see the doctor."

The citizens of Wolcott appealed to the Indiana State medical school, largest in the country. They wrote to every intern in every hospital in the state. They advertised in newspapers as far away as Chicago. They flew banners over football games reading, "Wolcott Needs a Doctor!" And they kept an office vacant, hoping to find a young physician to fill it.

On one occasion, the dean of the state medical school and a medical student came to answer anxious questions at a town meeting. As to the chance of getting a doctor, the student told them bluntly:

"I think its kind of poor. I think its not just poor for this town, but for many small towns across the nation that are trying to get physicians. It isn't money, and it is only partially what the community has to offer. The doctor is really no different from any other professional. My colleagues want better hours. Maybe it all sounds selfish, but a student can treat a hundred a day in Indianapolis or a hundred a day in this area. He just chooses to treat his hundred sick there. So, let me ask you: Why should a member of my class in medical school choose to come to this town?"

A man in the audience said, "One reason for coming here is that we have sick people here." The student did not answer.

The dean of the medical school tried to put the problem

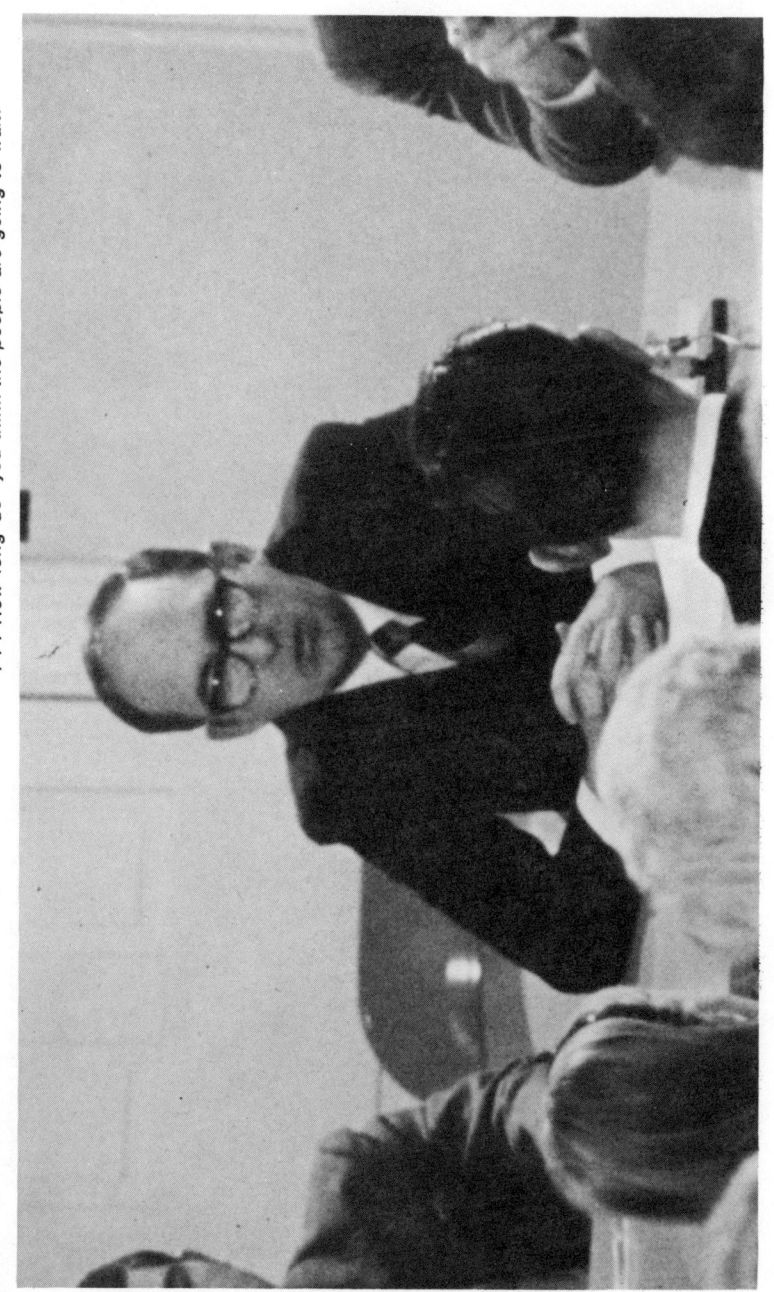

"... How long do you think the people are going to wait?"

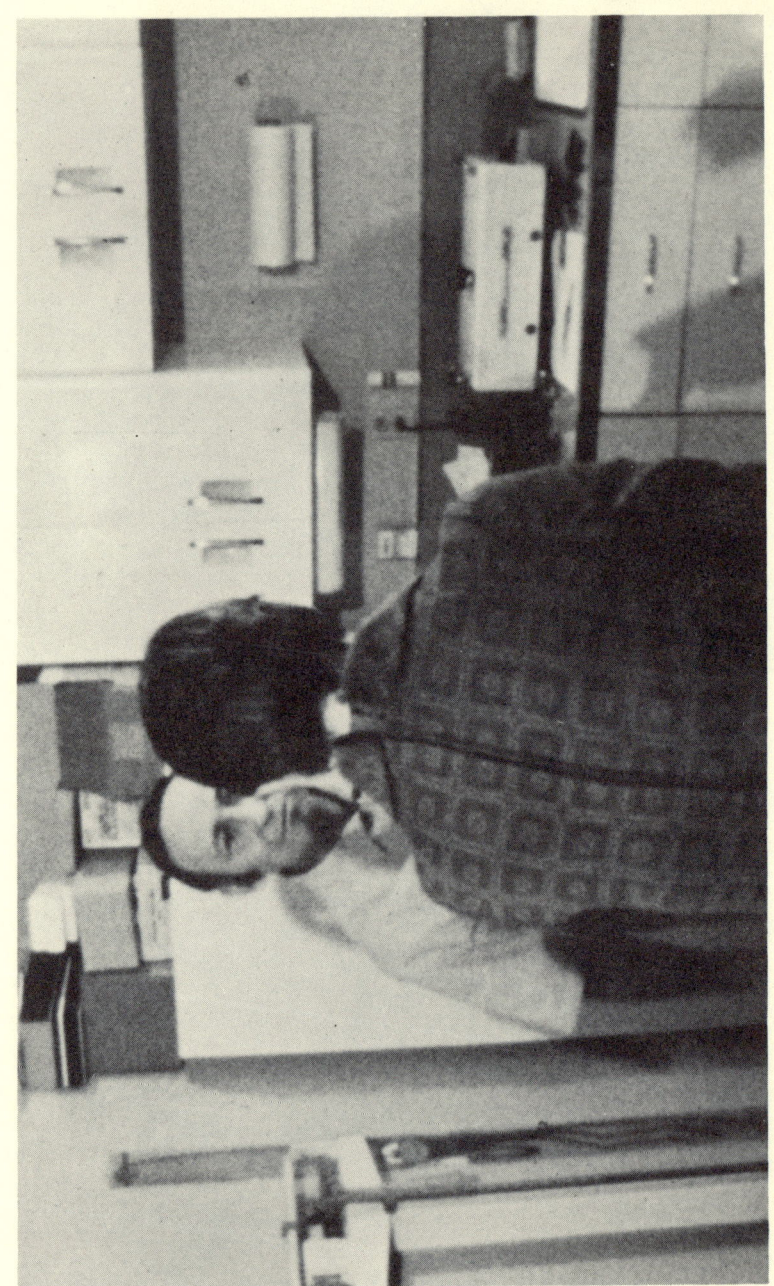

"What am I going to do for another doctor, George?"

in its broader context. "It's obvious that we have a rural problem and we have an urban problem, in this state and in most states. And although the cities have more doctors per population, there is a need for a lot more. I'm sure the people of this country and of this state are going to really put the pressure on us in medical education. But we have a situation that may get worse before it gets better."

Another man stood up from the audience. "How long do you think the people of Indiana, or the people of the United States, in the small areas, are going to wait? Do you think that they'll stand still? Or will they force something on the medical profession that the profession doesn't want?"

After two years without a doctor, Wolcott recently got one. The community is praying that he'll stay. Thousands of other "Wolcotts" still have none.

Some larger towns have doctors, but not enough. There is something poignant that happens when the neighborhood doctor quits. We saw that in Poughkeepsie, New York, a middle-class, medium-sized, mostly white city.

After fifteen years, Dr. George Kraus gave up his practice. One patient, receiving her final check-up, said, "I don't know why you'd do a thing like that. You know we've depended on you for all these years. What am I going to do for another doctor, George?"

But Dr. Kraus had had enough of eighty-hour weeks and twenty-four hour demands and years without a vacation—a fact of life for many American doctors who legitimately complain that they are vastly overworked. Dr. Kraus wanted now to return to public health. He tried hard to find someone to take over his practice.

"I offered it gratis to anyone that I thought might be capable of handling it, and unfortunately there was no one interested in it. This was difficult for me to understand because I have a fine, lucrative practice. But no younger men seem interested in taking it. They want to know whether they're going to work nights, weekends, holidays, whether they have to make house calls, whether they're going to have enough time off. And they also want to know how much money they're going to make in practice. Unfortunately, some of them even ask for a guarantee of a certain income.

"If what has occurred with me now in attempting to get a new physician continues this way, then certainly it's going to be harder in this community and other communities like it to get adequate medical care."

And that is only the problem of white, middle-class America!

* * *

Marianna, Arkansas: "Have You Any Money, Honey?"

Wolcott, Indiana, and Poughkeepsie, New York, have trouble getting a doctor for love or money. It's harder when there is little of either.

Lee County, in eastern Arkansas along the Mississippi, is what you mean when you talk of "rural poverty." Of its 21,000 inhabitants, a little more than half are black. When the larger farms were mechanized, tenants were pushed off the land and their tarpaper shacks bulldozed away. Average per capita income in 1966 was $1,039. The Blacks are not seething with resentment like those across the river in Mississippi. In fact, there is no civil rights organization in the whole county. Among the poor, running water is a scarcity, indoor toilets a dream, milk a rarity. What is well known is disease.

There are four doctors in Lee County, all white, all located in Marianna, the county seat. One is eighty-one years old and semi-retired. One is sixty and relatively inactive. One is a middle-aged woman who says that "the exchange of money is necessary to establish the proper relationship between doctor and patient." The youngest, in his early forties, has a "Wallace for President" button on his desk, segregated waiting rooms, and says "these people" spend all their money on whisky and cigarettes. And, for what help poor Blacks might get in Marianna, they mostly cannot come because they cannot pay the $10 to $25 for a ride into town.

In 1968, young Dr. Dan Blumenthal of St. Louis, full of enthusiasm and ideals, came to Lee County as a VISTA volunteer—the one and only VISTA doctor in the United

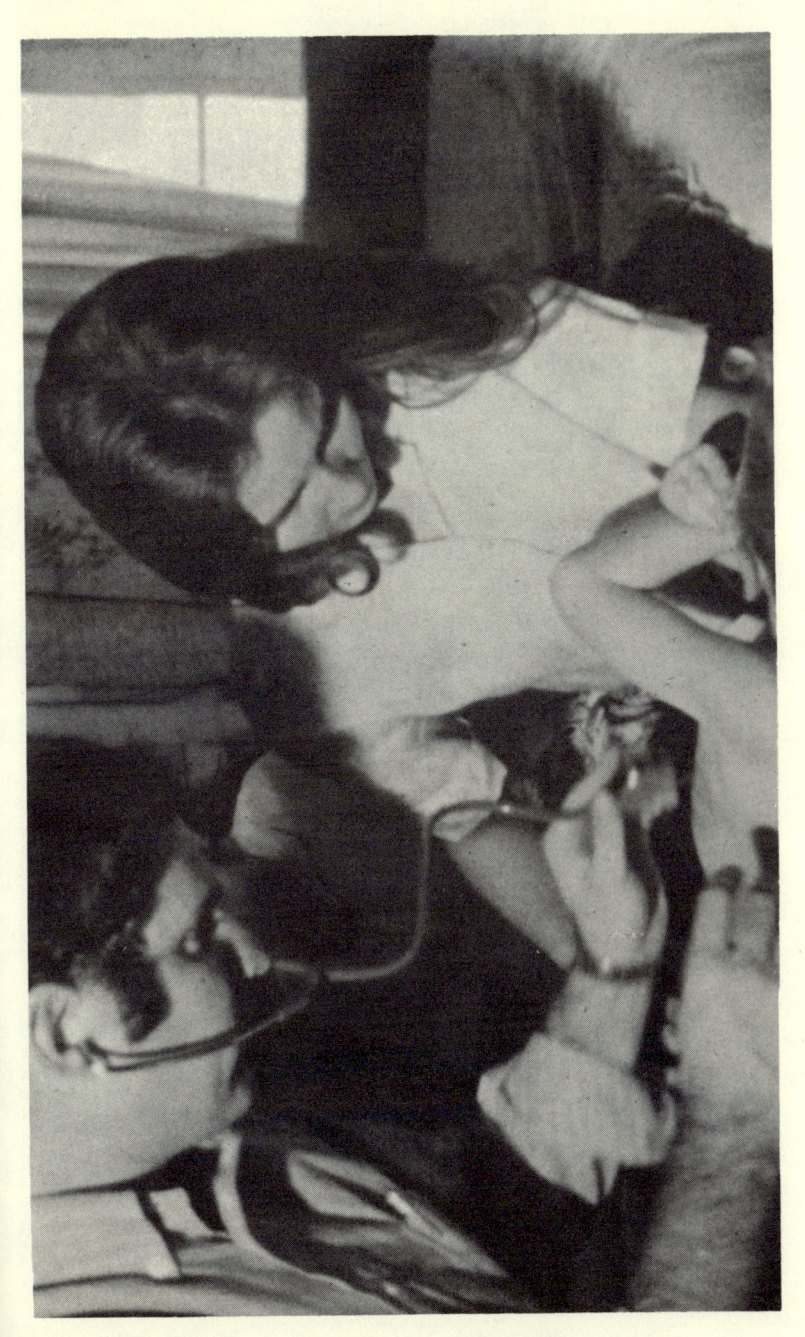

Medical care is still being picked by hand.

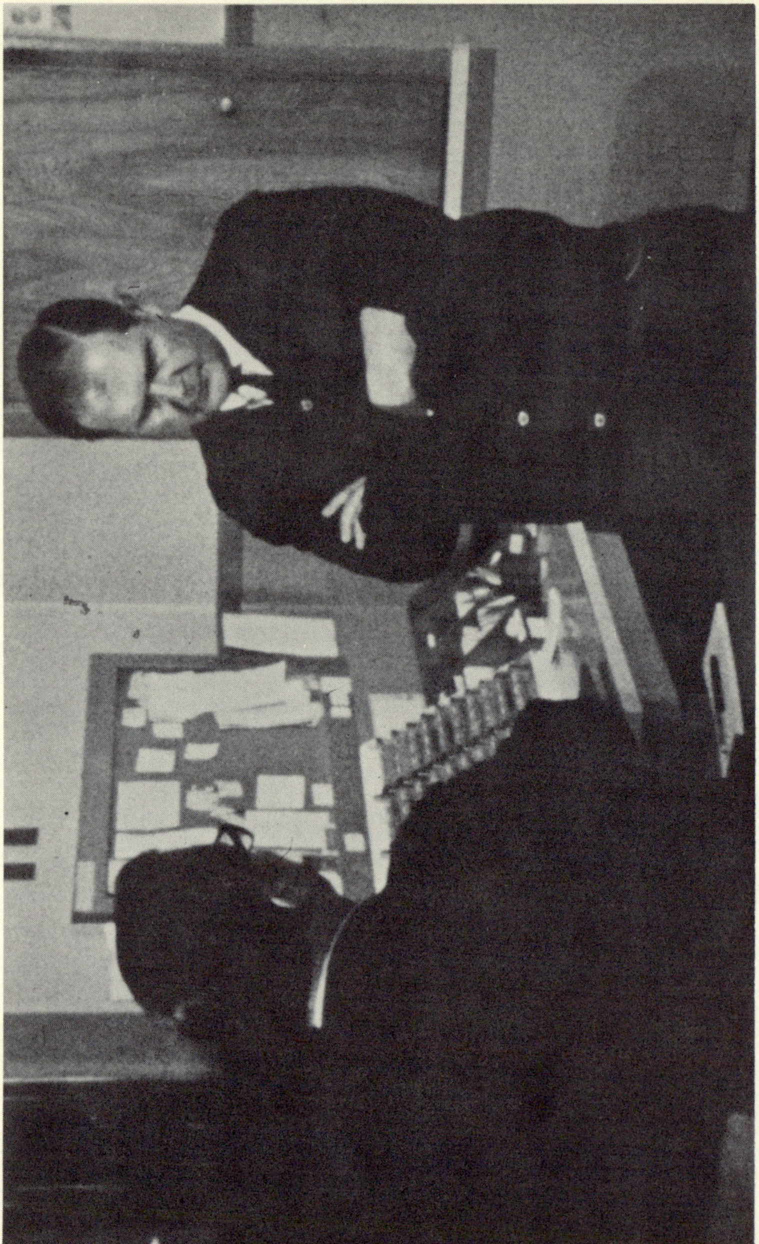

States—to practice medicine free for those who needed it most. He covered a hundred miles a day, six days a week, and felt the cold hostility of the establishment. He was refused the use of the local hospital (because he was not "engaged in the practice of private medicine," the board chairman said) and barred from the county medical society. Interviewed by George Herman, Dr. Blumenthal sketched this picture of health conditions in Lee County:

"In the rural areas the delivery of medical care is something that has made no progress whatever. Around here it has fallen way behind the progress in cotton picking and mechanized planting. Medical care is still being picked by hand. You see infectious disease. You see parasites that you might expect to see in Latin America but not in the United States. People stay sick. They go on with the same problems for year after year—the same aches and pains, the same headaches, the same arthritis. And they don't get treated.

"The health care, or lack of health care, the people receive in an area such as this leads to early death. Perhaps it's more than early death. It's early death following a lifetime of frustration and hopelessness and trying to do something about their health. People know that their health is bad. People suspect, I'm sure, that they're dying younger than they need to because they can't get the attention they need. And yet there's nothing they can do about it. It's just a hopeless feeling."

One day Correspondent Herman made the rounds with Dr. Blumenthal. In Marianna, they visited the family of Richard Griffin, twenty-two, unable to work regularly because of a back ailment. He has had it since he was fourteen, and it is still undiagnosed. His wife, Linda, is twenty-one. They had a three-month-old baby, and Dr. Blumenthal asked Griffin if they had any trouble finding someone to deliver the child.

"Yes, I did. While my wife was pregnant, she got sick all at once, and I thought she needed a doctor. I called a doctor, and he said he wouldn't see her. I called another doctor. He wouldn't see her. They said they had to have cash money

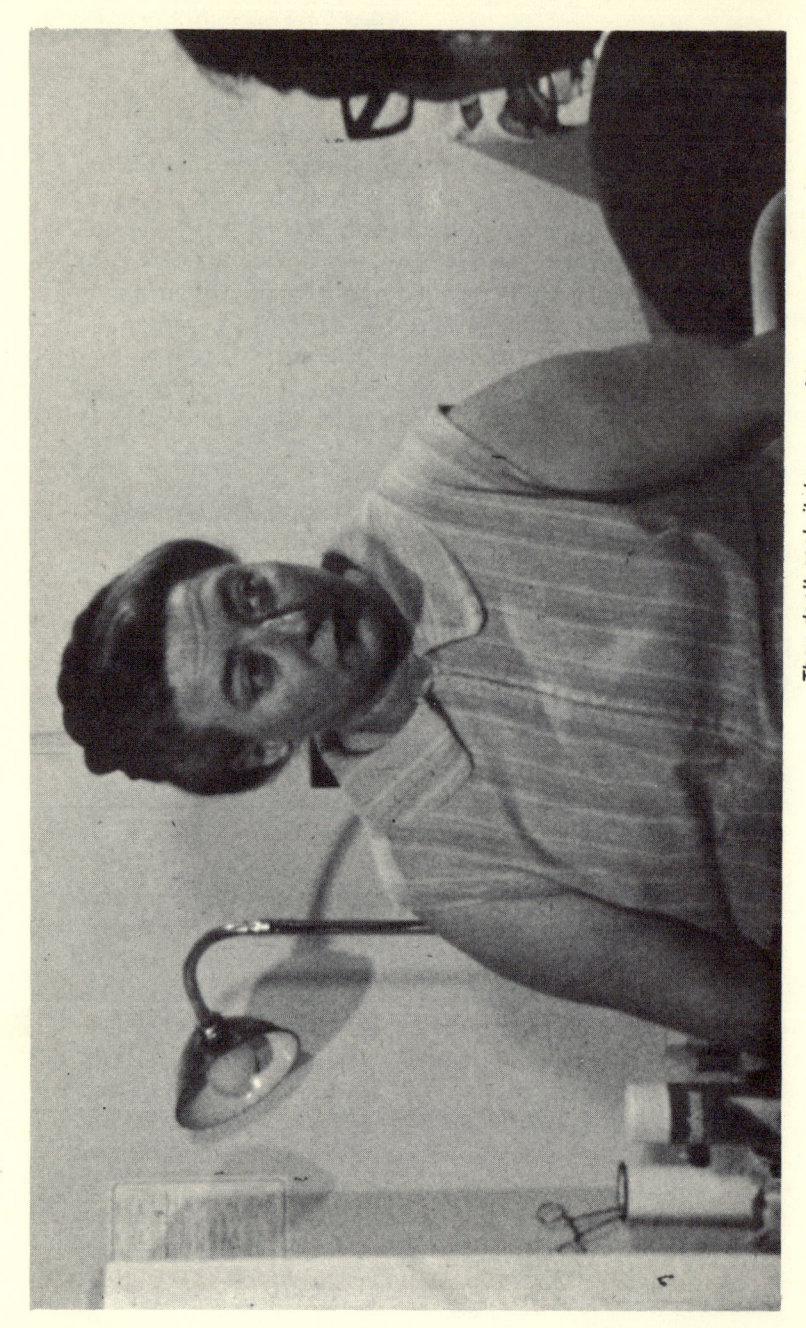

". . . They don't seek it because of ignorance or laziness."

before they could do it. So I called the doctor who delivered me when I was a baby. He said to bring cash money and he would take care of it. So I took my wife to one doctor here in Marianna, and she did take care of her. But in order for me to have my wife taken care of I had to get $25 in cash and write a hot check and let the doctor hold it. The baby was born and we had to rush the baby to the hospital in Little Rock. If we hadn't gotten over to Little Rock I don't think it would have lived."

There were others who talked of how hard it was to get medical assistance in Lee County:

"We've got people that's got to come as far as twenty or twenty-five miles to the doctor. Now, I think the doctors is really doing their best. But they just is overloaded. And these people gotta come as far as twenty or twenty-five miles when they pay four or five dollars to come to the house. Then they don't have the money to pay the doctor or to buy medicine. And we've got lots of people in Lee County that is going lackin' for medical care. . . . "

"We can't find doctors on a Thursday. You all ought to know that you can't get a doctor here on Thursday evening out at the hospital when you get ready. And you can't hardly get one to come to the country to make a call in the country. . . . "

"I've taken a lady right to the office and stayed there until she waited on her, until she examined her. And before she put a hand on her, she said, 'Do you have any money, honey?' And the lady told her she had some. The doctor said she wanted to know where she was goin' to get the money from. If you ain't got no money, you don't see no doctor. You just have to suffer it out. . . . "

Lee County does have some medical facilities. In the building that used to be the county jail, there is a public health office. It supervises the thirteen midwives who deliver babies in the county. There is one public health nurse. Mrs. Helen Whitworth has been that nurse since 1937. She says that she needs four more nurses to meet public health standards. She

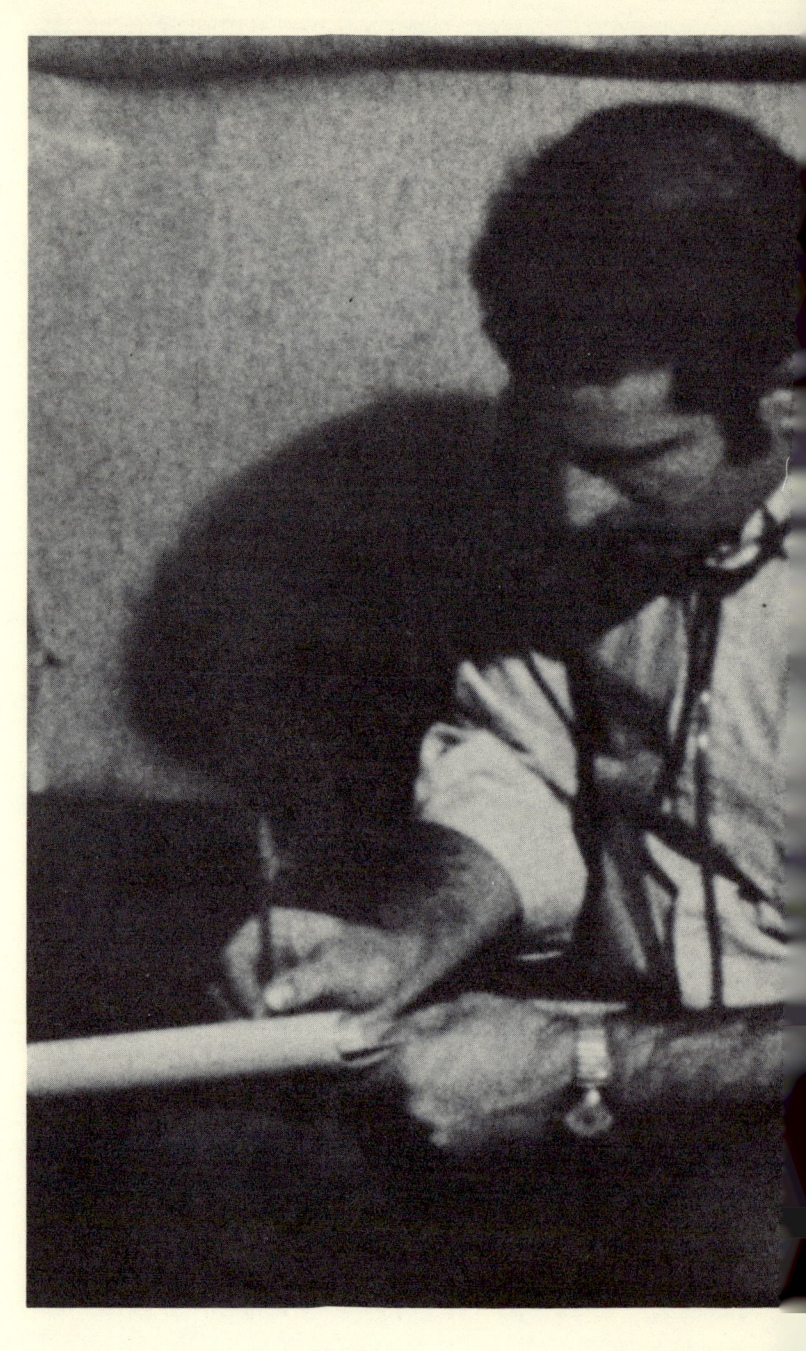

"Some new way is

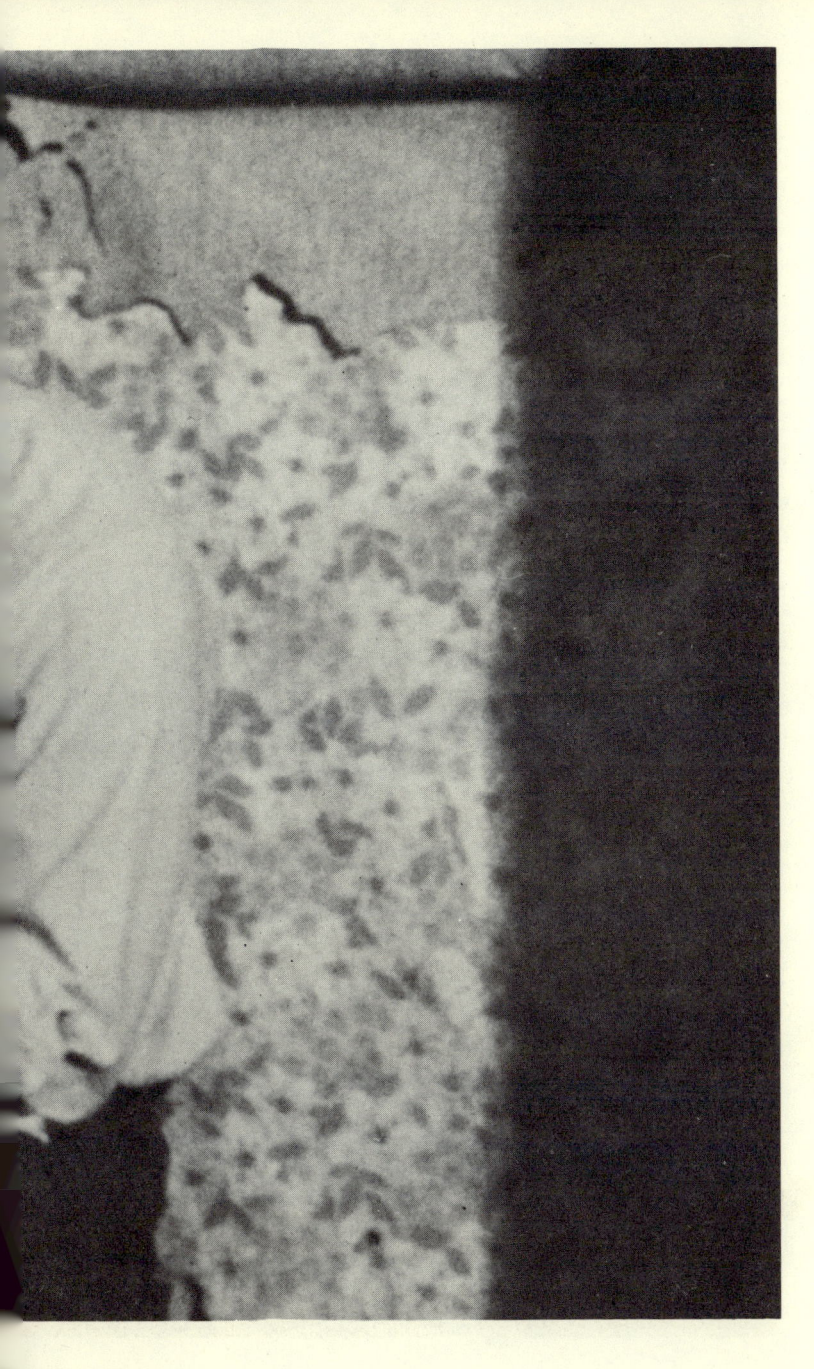

ve to be found."

needs many more incubators to combat an infant death rate that compares with that of Paraguay.

There is one hospital with twenty-seven beds. It has a modern, fully equipped operating room but no surgeon. It has a complete laboratory but no one trained to read X-rays.

Paul Benham, Jr., insurance agent and a power in the county, is chairman of the hospital board. He said, "We think that the hospital is adequate, physically. We do need professional help—nurses and doctors. But we have nothing to apologize for, nothing to hide in this community so far as the professional services rendered by members of our medical society are concerned. They're hard-working people; they work twenty-four hours a day, seven days a week. And I resent uninformed people who have never been in our community, who know nothing of our problems, and only print or talk about the bad side. We take care of our people."

Mr. Benham's view that "we take care of our people" is supported by the four doctors of Marianna. Dr. Mac McClendon, eighty-one years old, says, "I've been practicing medicine here for fifty-three years, and I never seen anybody yet that couldn't get a doctor if they needed one." Dr. Elizabeth Fields says, "They get adequate medical care if they come seeking it. So many times they're sick and they don't seek it because of ignorance or laziness." And she denied that she had ever turned anyone away for lack of money.

There is dispute about whether poor people get turned away but no dispute about the hundreds who never get close enough to the doctor's office to find out if they will be turned away. Young Dr. Blumenthal continued bringing free medicine to the poor on his exhausting daily rounds until his VISTA tour was over. Then he looked back and said that what he had done was "no more than even a drop in the bucket."

"There aren't enough doctors," he said. "People can't afford to see the doctor. Transportation is bad. People can't get in to see the doctor. They can't afford to see the doctor. They don't get examined. They don't get preventive medicine. They don't get follow-up on their acute problems. And their health is bad. Certainly there are many hundreds of areas like this

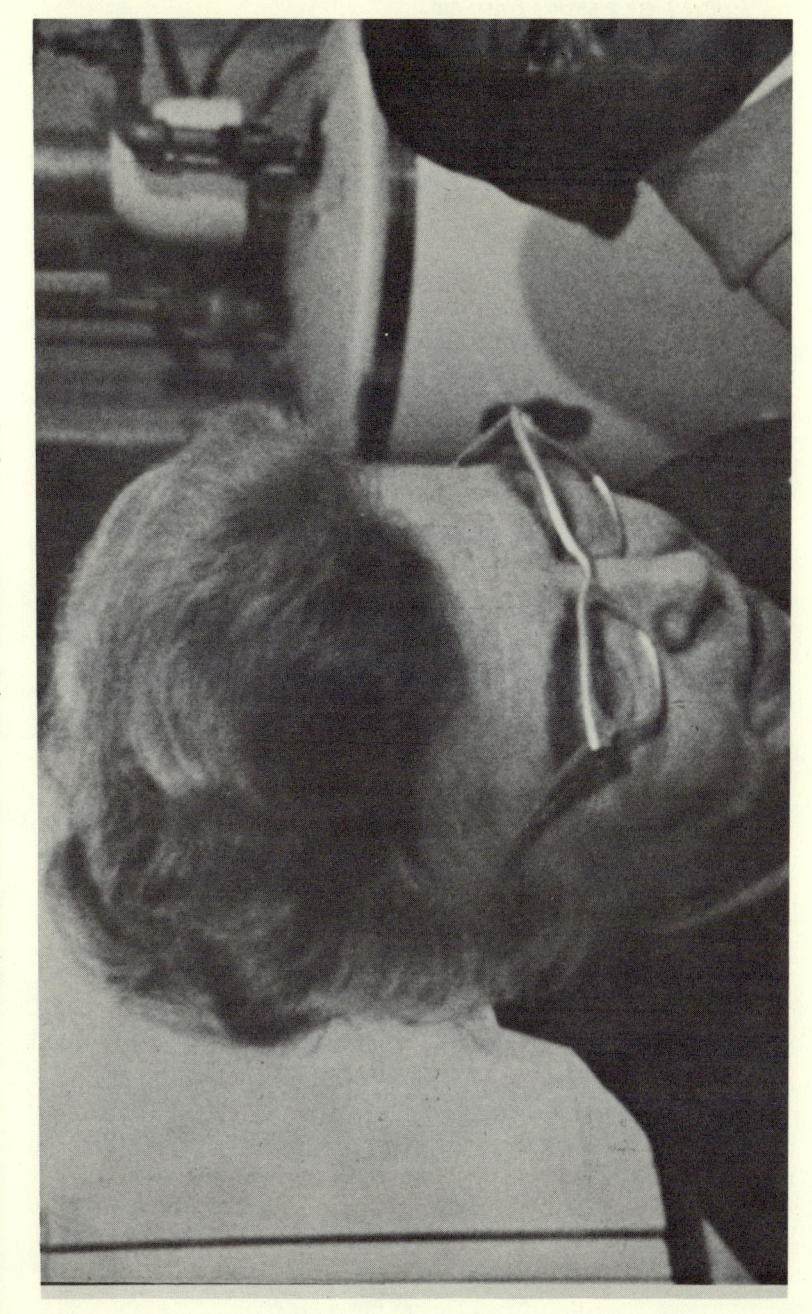

... an infant death rate that compares with that of Paraguay.

around the country where these problems cannot be solved by the traditional means of delivering health care. Some new way is going to have to be found to deliver health care to people in areas like this."

* * *

Chicago, Illinois: Welfare Doctor, Welfare Patient

Chicago is the medical capital of America. It is the headquarters of the American Medical Association, with an annual budget of $34 million. Chicago has eighty hospitals and five medical schools. But in the West Side ghetto, with 300,000 people and disease rates three to four times the national average, people have to travel miles and wait for hours for access to the one charity hospital that must take them in—Cook County, the nation's largest general hospital.

Cook County, on the day of our visit, was bursting at the seams. More than a thousand persons daily crowd into its registration and emergency room for treatment. They are not necessarily emergency cases, but for many it is the only way to see a doctor. Many, discouraged by the wait, leave before they are attended. Others, who need a hospital bed, are sent home because no hospital bed is available. For those who are admitted, there may be waits of three to four hours for X-rays, even in emergencies. They are crowded into medical wards where there is one registered nurse for a hundred patients. Of those admitted, one out of every six dies.

Those who run Cook County Hospital grieve about the situation but have no solution. CBS News witnessed one frustrated consultation that must have happened hundreds of times. Dr. Hunter Cutting, director of medicine, talked to Dr. Jeb Boswell, director of admissions, estimating that he had one bed for every three persons needing a bed.

"Listen, is there anything we can do because we have six beds left in medicine, and there are a lot of them out there?"

Dr. Boswell said, "Well, you're going to get about seventy or eighty admissions today. And I think our standing agreement is that if you don't have beds in medicine, you send them off to general surgery."

Dr. Boswell went on, "This may be the night. We don't have enough technicians to give blood counts. We can't give them blood chemistries. We have this turnaround time in X-ray. We take a look at the X-ray delay times and say, 'Well it's better that they get under treatment without an X-ray than to keep them down there an additional three or four hours.' That is for emergency X-rays."

Dr. Cutting left him, muttering, "I don't know, frankly, where we're going to put that crowd out there."

The crowd "out there" in the receiving room was not as big as it could have been. Many from the West Side ghetto are reluctant to go to Cook County, even in dire need. They would prefer to go to a neighborhood doctor, but there are few neighborhood doctors in the ghetto. There are empty offices of physicians and surgeons who have long since left for richer territory. We found more doctors in one medical office building in the comfortable North Side than in the entire West Side ghetto.

Dr. Jean Bernier is one of the few who stayed, and he is branded by many of his colleagues with the epithet, "welfare doctor." Dr. Bernier often sees more patients in a day than his colleagues see in a week—as many as 150 in a twelve-hour day. And he told us how it is to be a "welfare doctor."

"You get complaints from organizations. You get complaints from your own physician friends. You get complaints from the hospitals. I'm afraid the doctors and hospitals need more education about the problems. For example, when you bring a patient to the hospital, they say, 'Well, here's Bernier with another welfare patient!' In other words, like it was something else, you know. Well, sometimes they are a little different because they're a little dirty. They're all alone and they haven't been able to wash themselves. They're senile. They may be a little more of a problem. But they need hospital care, and you can't send everybody to County. Many times you can't send people to County because they won't go. I've seen people die because they refused to go to County."

There are few hospitals that will take the poor, and there are few Dr. Berniers to try to send them. Frank Brown is

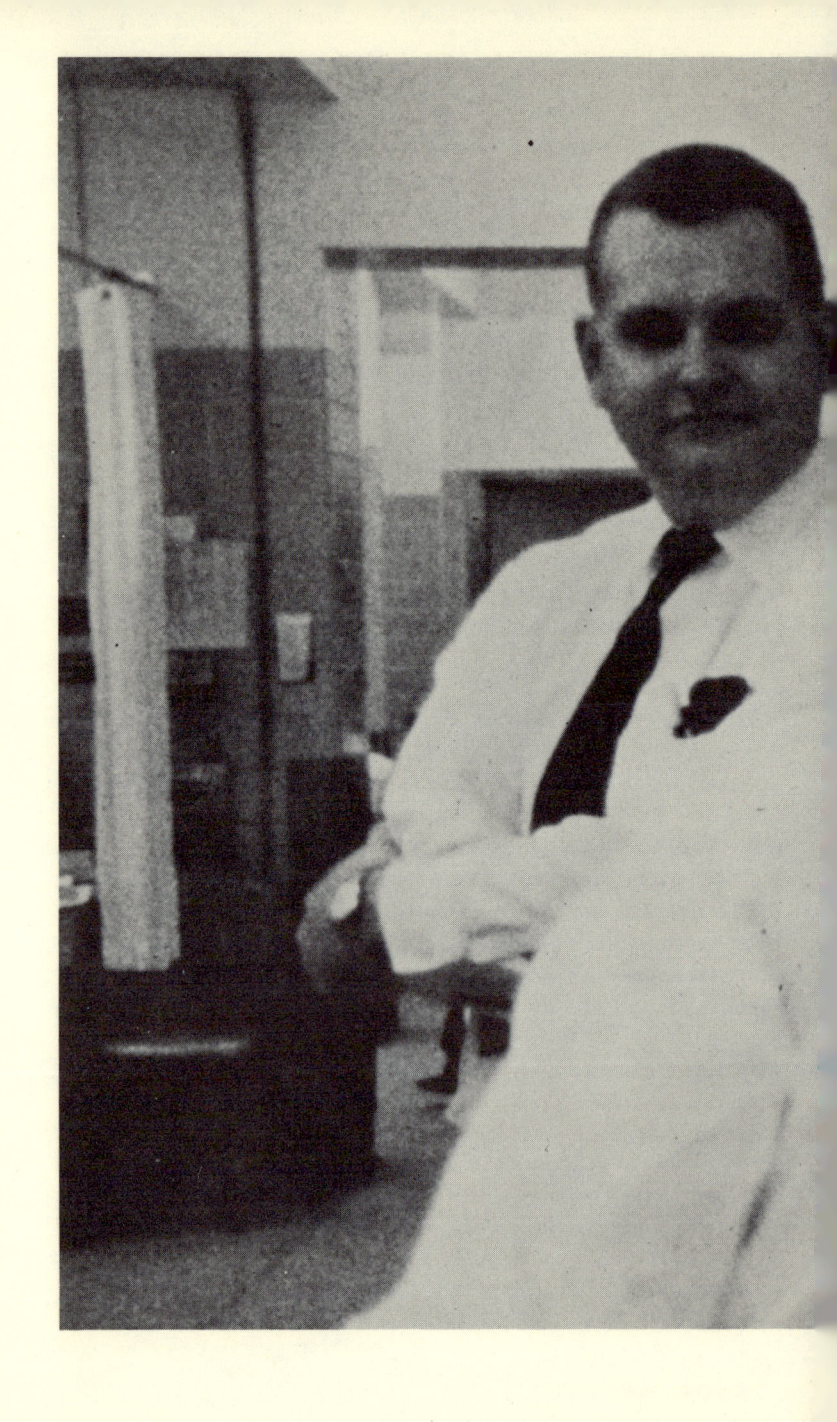

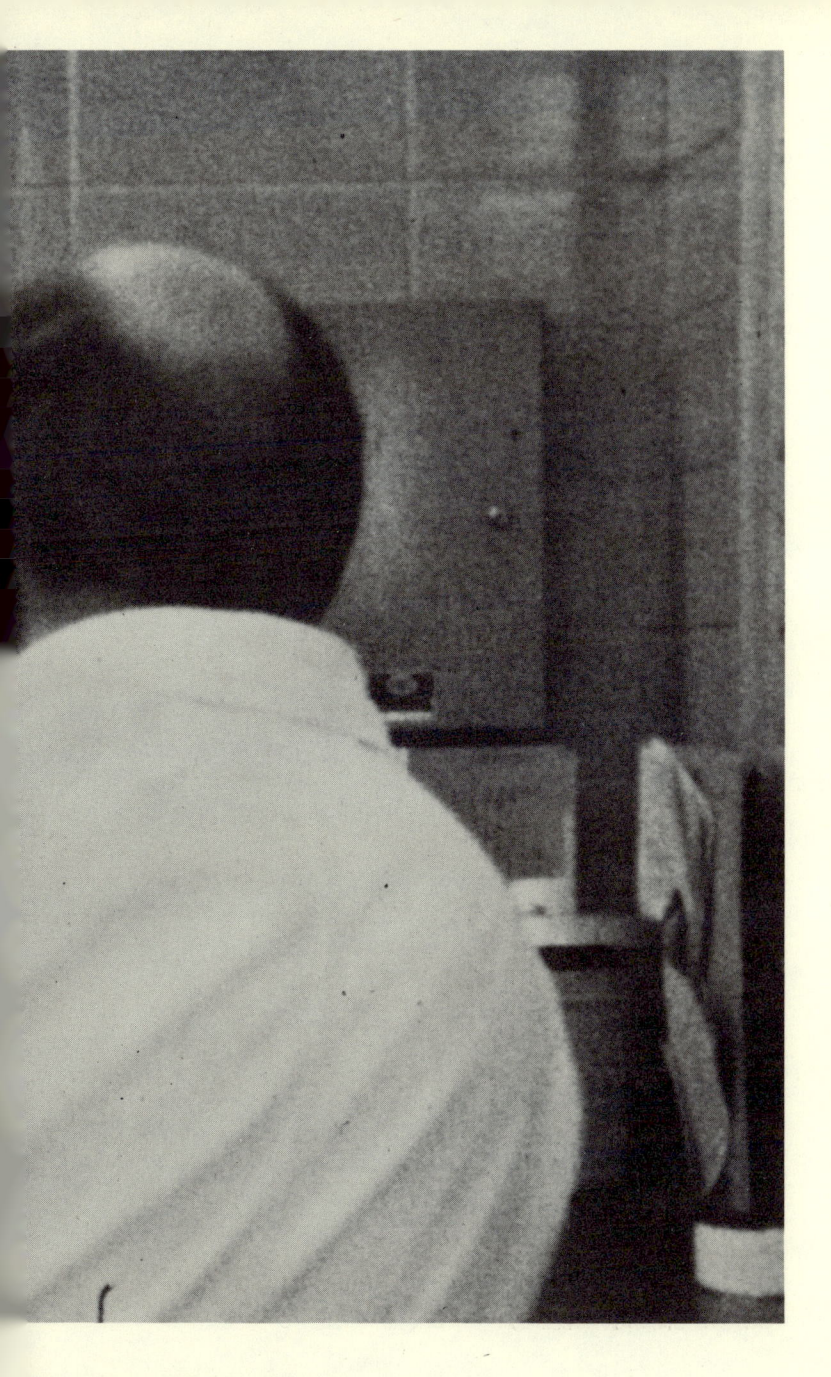

"This may be the night!"

a community health worker in Kenwood-Oakland, a community that has one doctor for every 15,000 people—less than one-tenth the national average. Brown became a health worker when his daughter died because he couldn't get her into a nearby hospital in time to save her.

CBS News was present when Brown called the welfare office from the home of an elderly woman, Mrs. Ivory Montgomery, whose legs were paining her from the hips down. Brown's end of the conversation went like this:

"Well, I don't know what happened. Only thing I know is that she can't walk and she needs a doctor. You know of no doctor who will come into the home? Doesn't public aid have working agreements with doctors where doctors will come to see patients who can't get about? You'll check with the medical department? The only thing I am interested in is that the lady is very sick and trying to get a doctor to see her. . . .

"Let me ask you this—isn't it the obligation of public assistance to send in medical help when a person is quite ill? She needs to see a doctor now—right now! You know, I've been calling for about an hour-and-a-half and, you know, everyone has the same story that the doctor just won't come out. . . . "

The doctor did not come to Mrs. Montgomery that day. Nor did an ambulance come to the home of Mrs. Laura Hayes, whom Brown found with a doctor's note saying that she needed immediate hospitalization. Nor did any help come in time to two other homes, where persons were found dead.

"We're already a sick society," says Brown, "and we'll become a sicker society simply because people just don't care. They're more interested in perpetuating the wars, more interested in getting to the moon. They just aren't interested in people's health. I've been in homes where people are ill to the point where they need to be hospitalized, and hospitals will tell you that they're filled to capacity. There's no room. That's how people get to feel de-humanized. . . . "

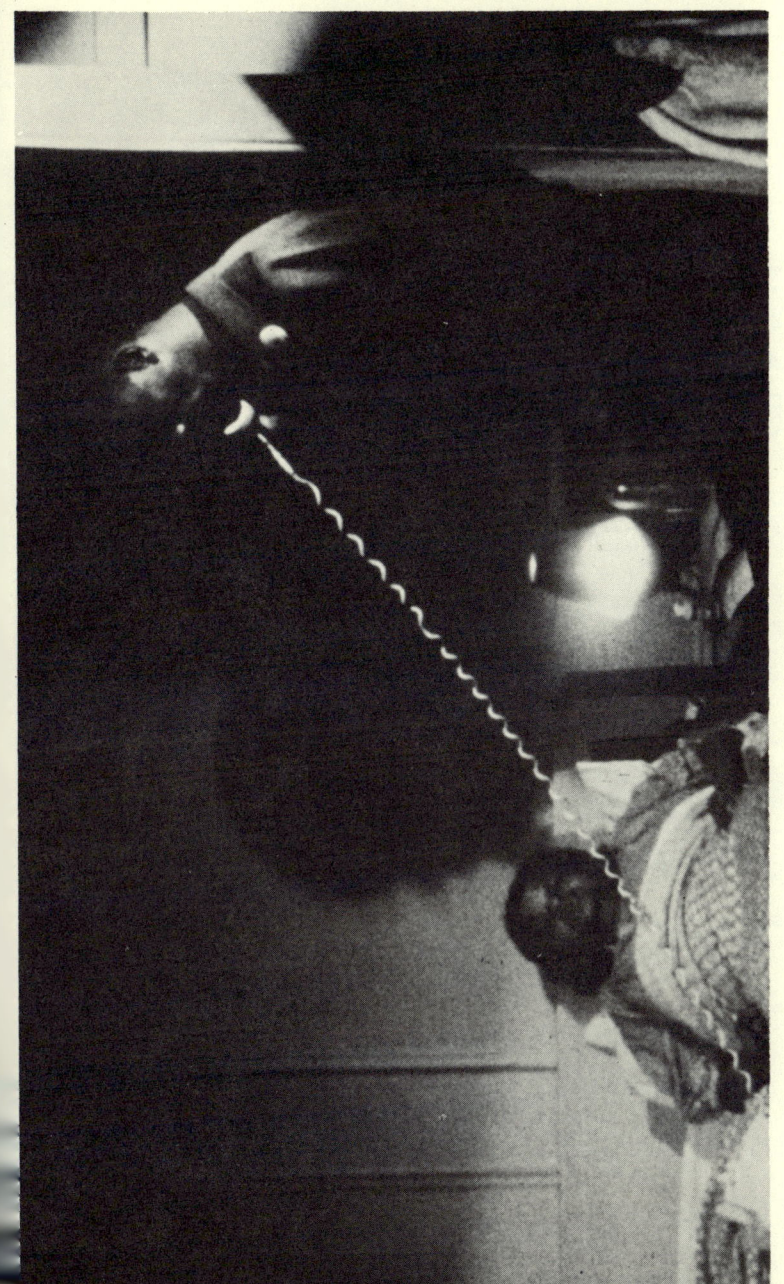

"She needs to see a doctor now—right now!"

CHAPTER III
THE "CORNER GROCERY" HOSPITAL

At Mt. Zion Hospital in San Francisco, one day in 1970 Alex Freedman checked in for a hernia operation, and CBS News checked in with him. Alex Freedman is no celebrity, and there was nothing especially newsworthy about his operation. The fifty-five-year-old novelty wholesaler, occupying one of 1.7 million beds in one of 7,000 hospitals that represent an investment of $28 billion, was simply our Mr. Average American Patient.

Alex Freedman was starting an experience that would be simple surgically, complicated financially.

From the moment Mr. Freedman entered the hospital, his charges began. Before going to his room, three blood samples and a urine sample were taken. The specimens were sent to the laboratory for a series of tests. The most elaborate is a chemical profile, performed on an automatic analyzer. These tests, required for all patients, are marked up above cost to help pay for deficits elsewhere. Charge to Mr. Freedman—$27.

Soon after arrival in his semi-private room, nursing service began. Cost—$28.18 daily, a part of the daily room charge of $71.50 daily. That room charge covered several services, including $6.37 for administrative costs, $6.30 for meals, $4.66 for house medical staff, $3.97 for medical records, $3.48 for depreciation, $2.09 for maintenance, $1.99 for laundry, $1.05 for social service, $4.66 for housekeeping, and $8.75 for "gain," meaning mark-up.

At the end of the first day, Mr. Freedman owed $99.75, including $71.50 for his room, $27 for laboratory and $1.25 for catheters.

His surgeon stopped in to see him and told him that everything was ready for the operation next day. Next morning at 7:30 Mr. Freedman was wheeled into the operating room. His hernia operation lasted an hour-and-a-half. The use of the operating room and its staff cost him $190.85. A routine biopsy to check for possible malignancy cost $22. The day of his operation cost him $302.60, including $71.50 for his hospital room, $190.85 for the operating room, $22 for biopsy, $9 for intravenous feeding, $9.25 for drugs.

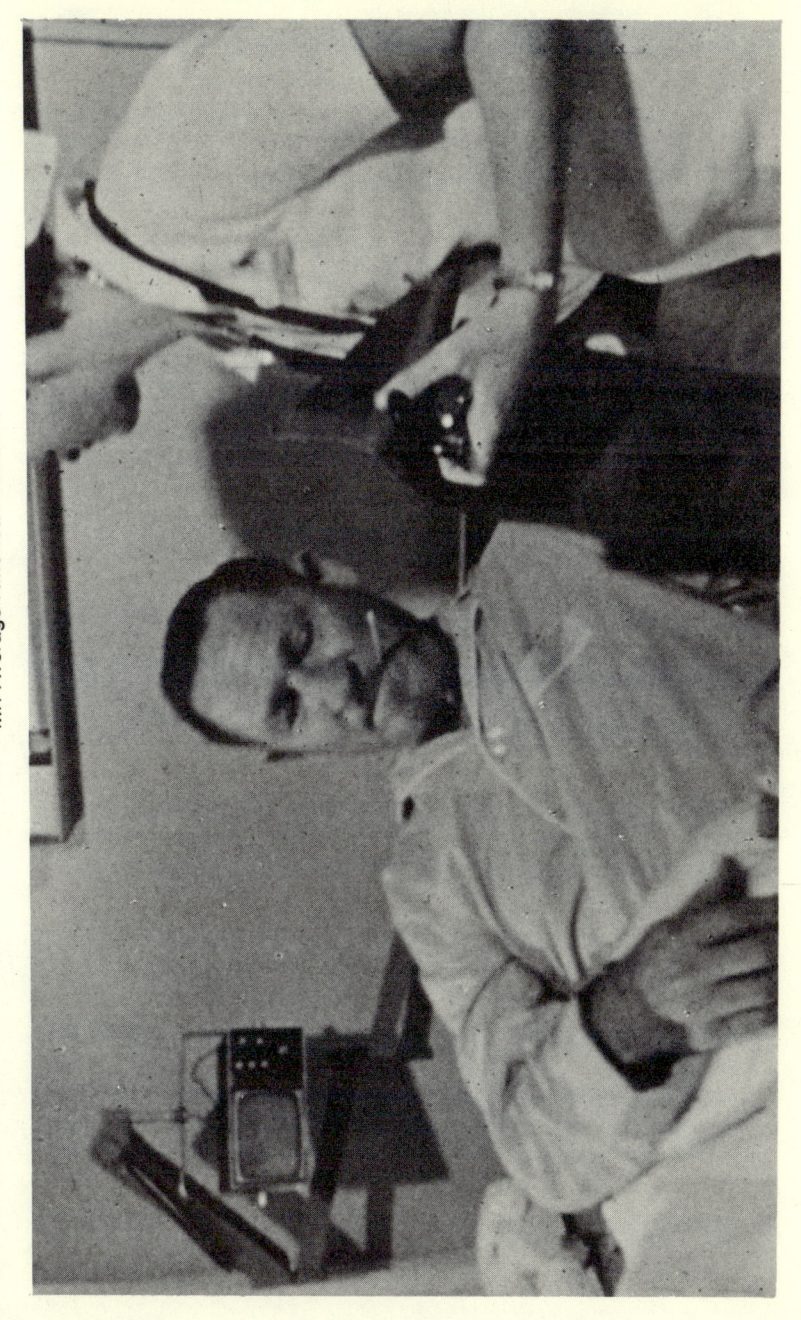

Mr. Average American Patient.

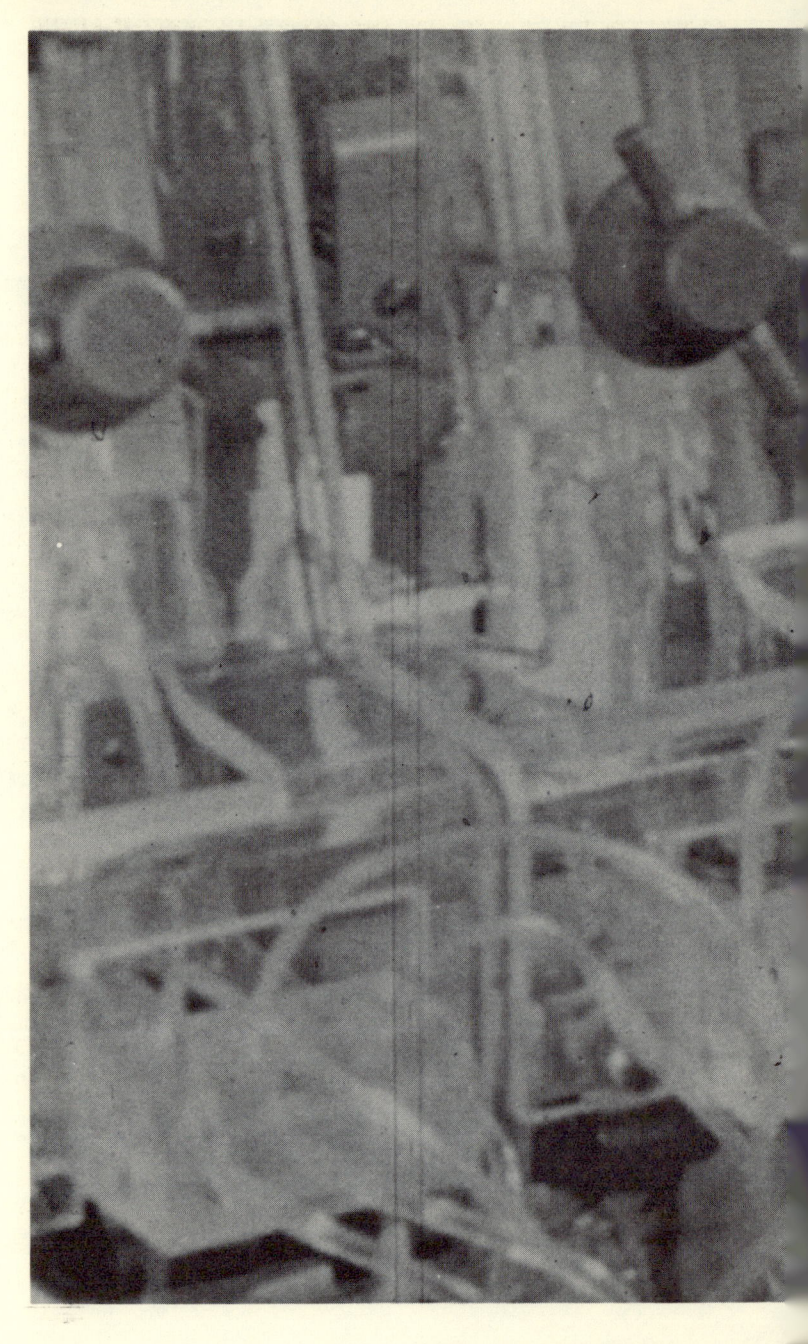

The most elaborate blood test—a c

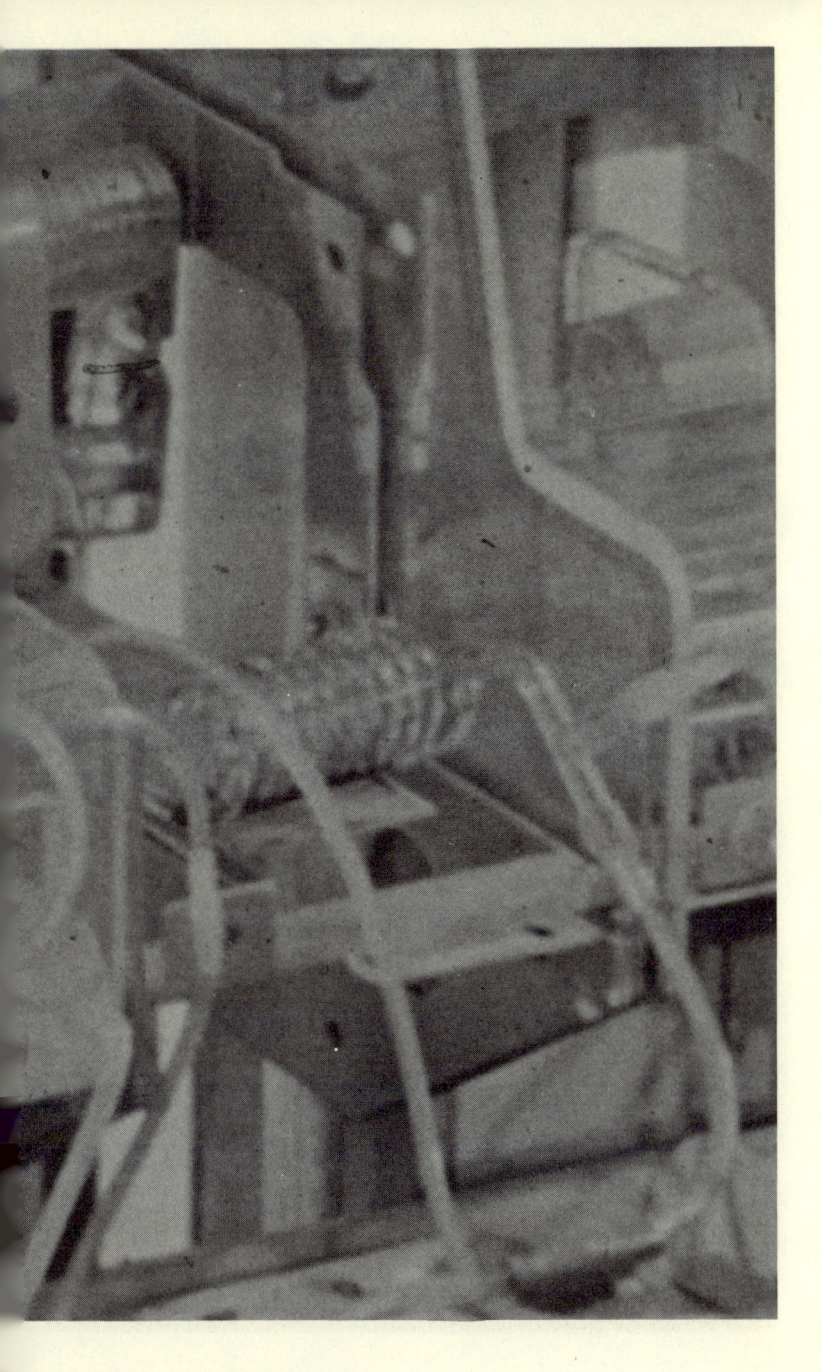

performed on an automatic analyzer.

THE HOSPITAL AND THE CASH REGISTER

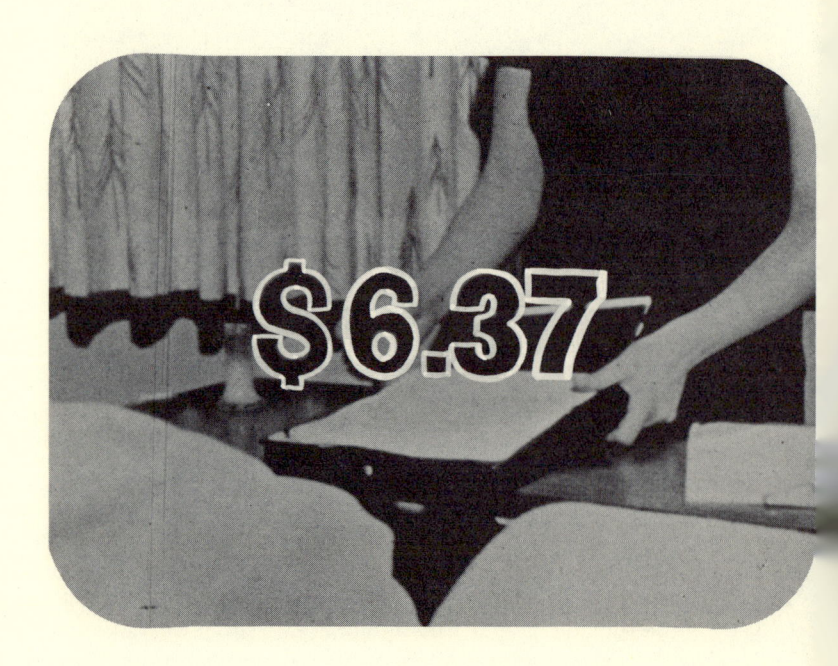

$6.37

$6.30

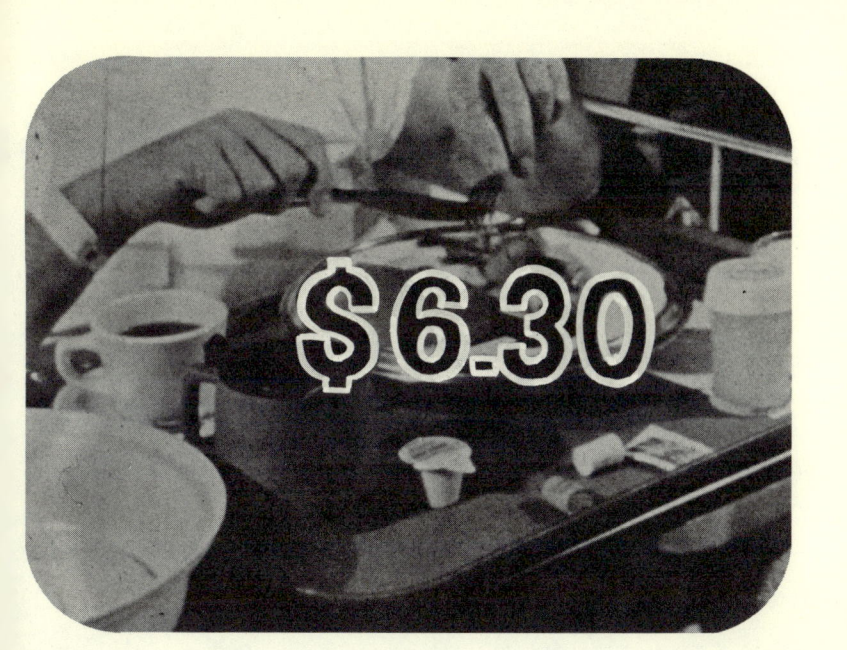

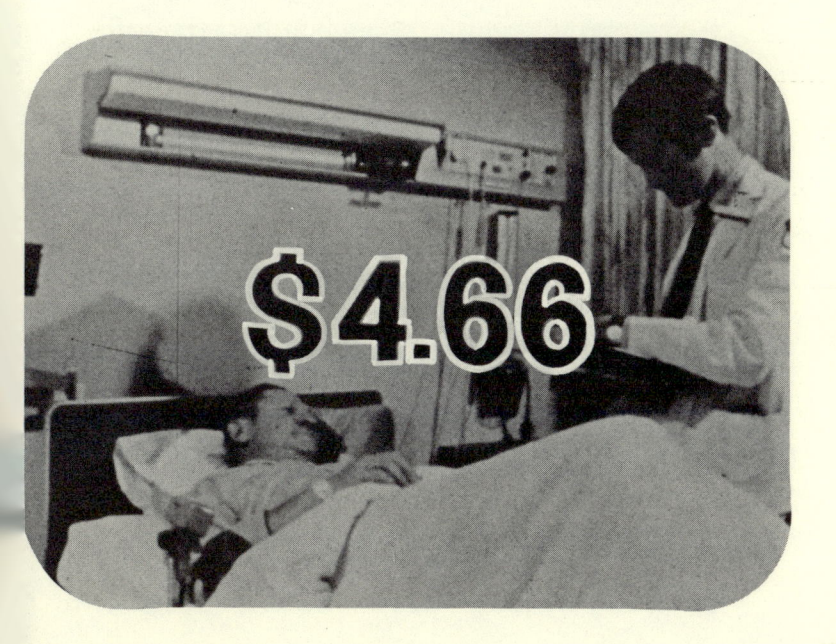

$4.66

$3.97

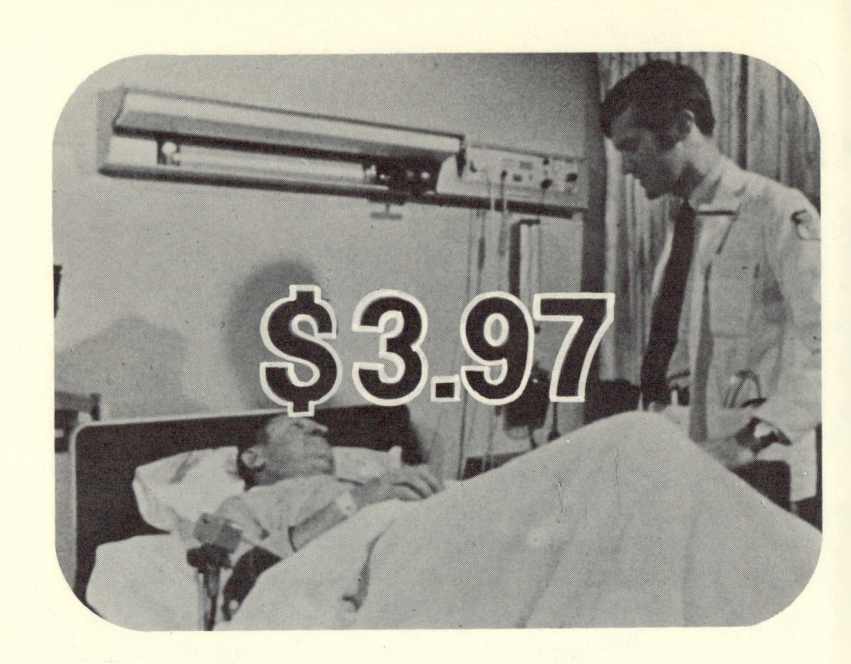

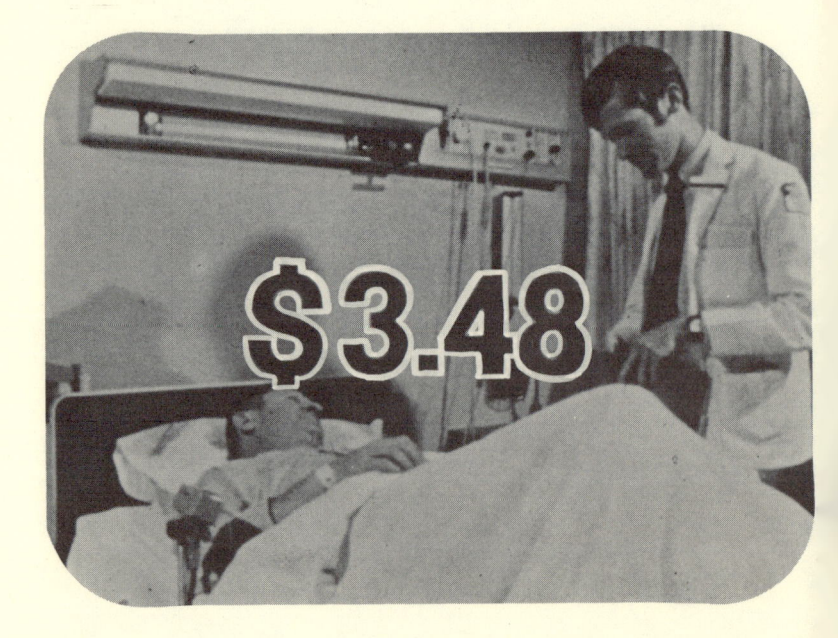

$3.48

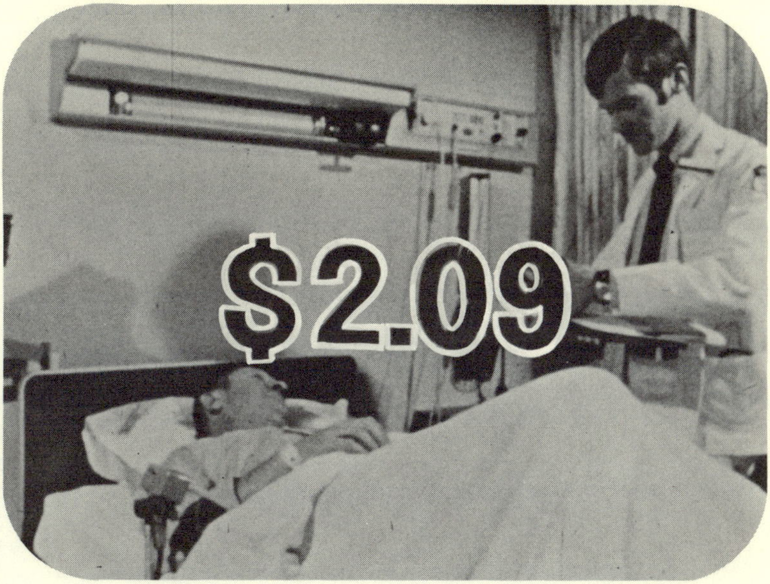
$2.09

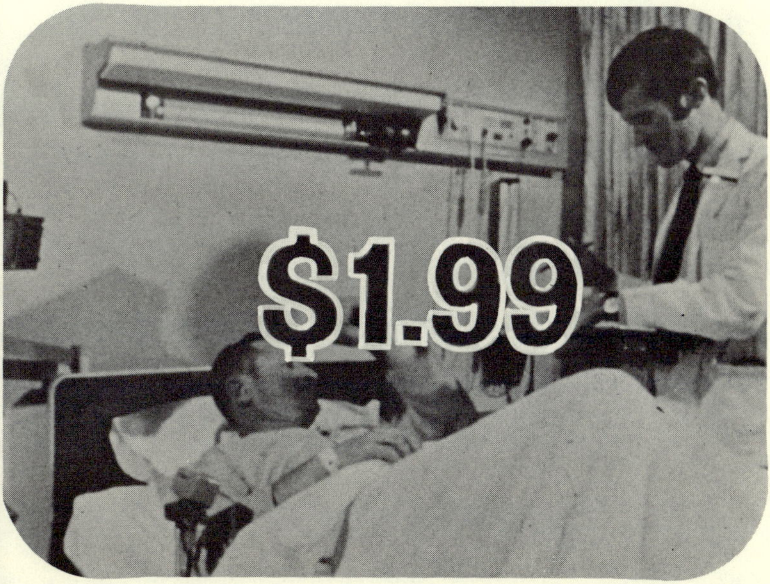
$1.99

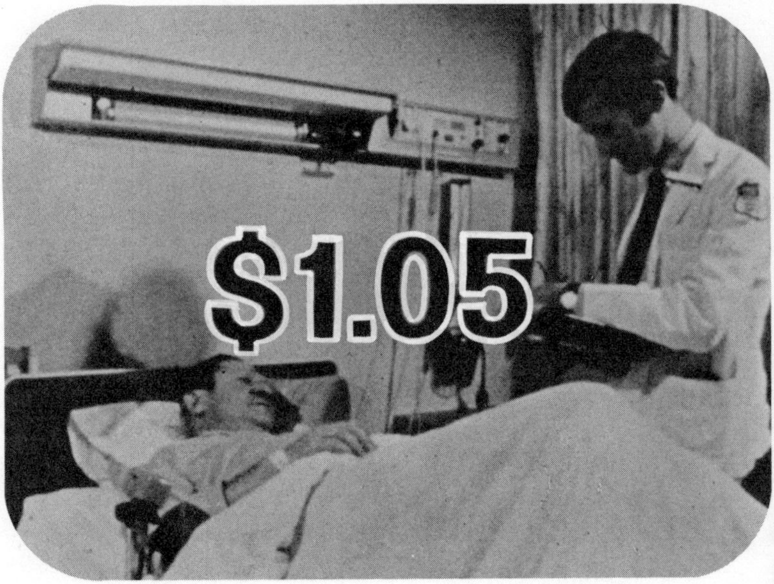
$1.05

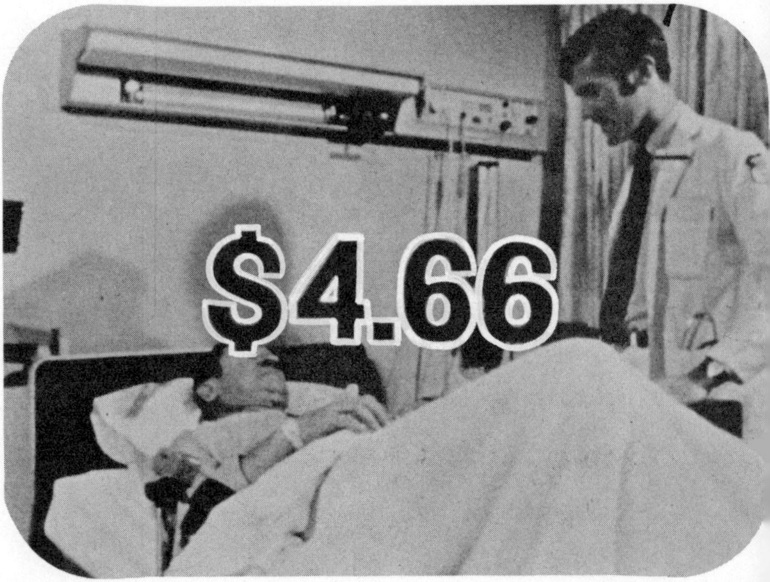
$4.66

$8.75

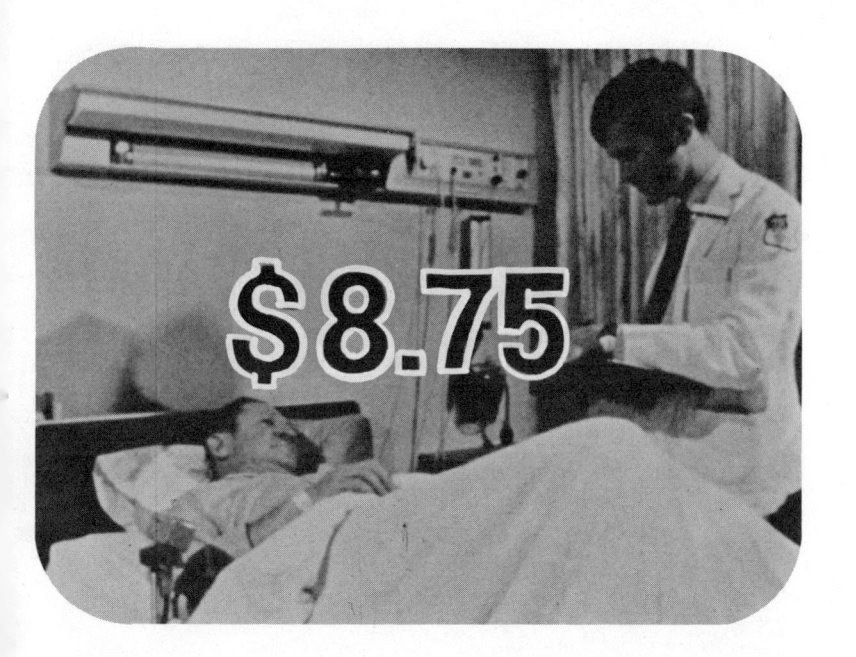

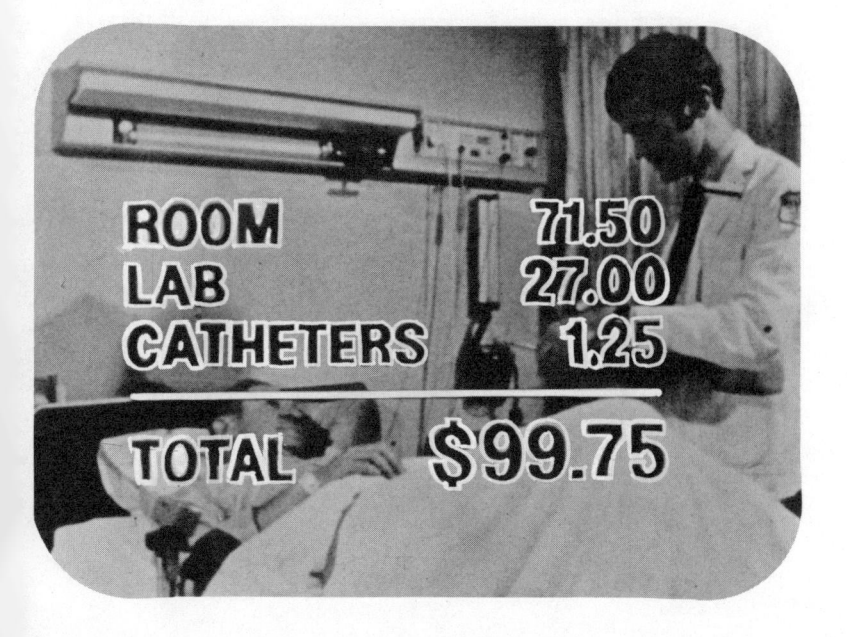

ROOM	71.50
LAB	27.00
CATHETERS	1.25
TOTAL	**$99.75**

$190.85

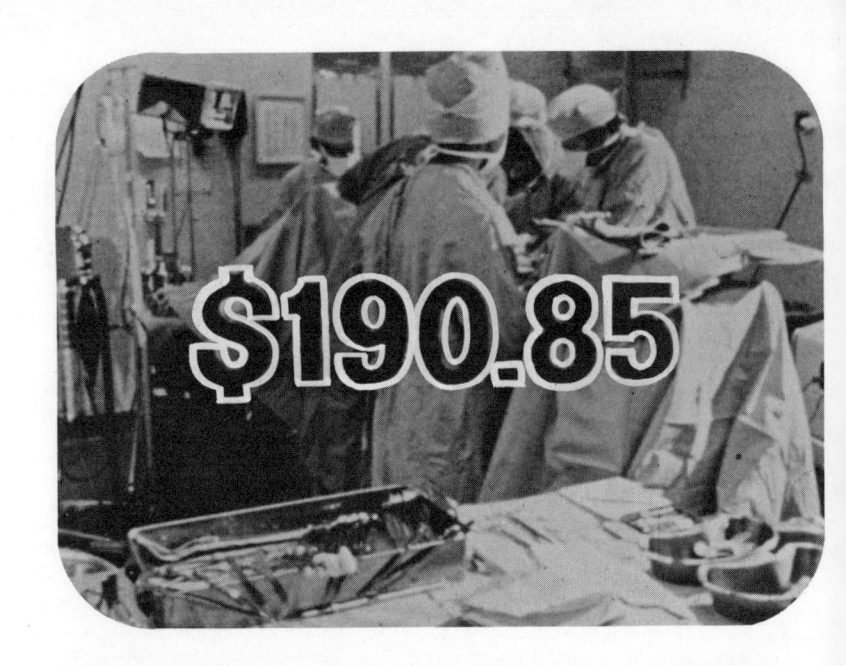

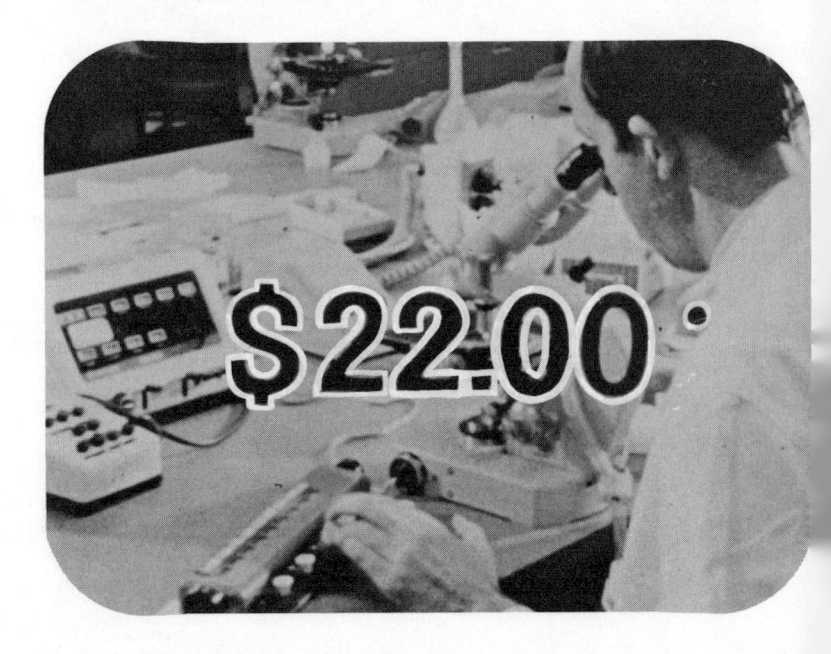

$22.00

ROOM	71.50
OPER. RM.	190.85
BIOPSY	22.00
INTRAVENOUS	9.00
DRUGS	9.25
TOTAL	**$302.60**

HOSPITAL	641.35
SURGEON	300.00
ANESTHETIST	76.50
TOTAL	**$1,017.85**

DON'T GET SICK IN AMERICA

On the fifth day Mr. Freedman was ready to go home. At the cashier's office he was presented with a bill for $616.35, which was not the final bill. He would be advised within ten days of what more he owed. The balance brought his hospital bill to $641.35. Then came the surgeon's bill for $300 and the anesthetist's bill for $76.50. Mr. Freedman's hernia operation and five days in the hospital had cost him a total of $1,017.85—to be paid by him since he had no health insurance.

To repeat, there was nothing unusual about Mr. Freedman, his operation or his bill. He had simply shared the experience of millions of Americans—the explosion of hospital costs, rising five times as fast as the cost of living, which has been rising fast enough. Ten years before, Mr. Freedman's thousand-dollar operation would have cost him half as much. Ten years later, unless something happens it could cost him more than twice as much.

In early 1970, an average hospital day nationally cost about $70. But it was much higher in big cities—$110 in New York, $103 in Boston, $90 in Chicago, $88 in Minneapolis, $90 in New Orleans, and $117 in Los Angeles. Unless something drastic happens, the national average will be $98 by 1973. At a hearing of the Senate Finance Committee, Senator Abraham Ribicoff, former secretary of HEW, raised the staggering possibility of $1,000 a day for hospital care in large cities by 1980.

When you ask why hospital prices are out-pacing virtually every other form of inflation, you get some standard answers. First, the belated catch-up in sub-standard wages—and labor represents seventy percent of a hospital's costs. Once among the country's most underpaid employees, with wages as low as thirty-five cents an hour in some parts of the South, hospital employees have raised their standards by unionization and strikes, aided by minimum-wage requirements.

Secondly, the technological revolution, resulting in a fabulously expensive array of new medical hardware, with cost spread among patients whether or not they use it. Mr. Freedman did not use but helped to pay for Mt. Zion's kidney

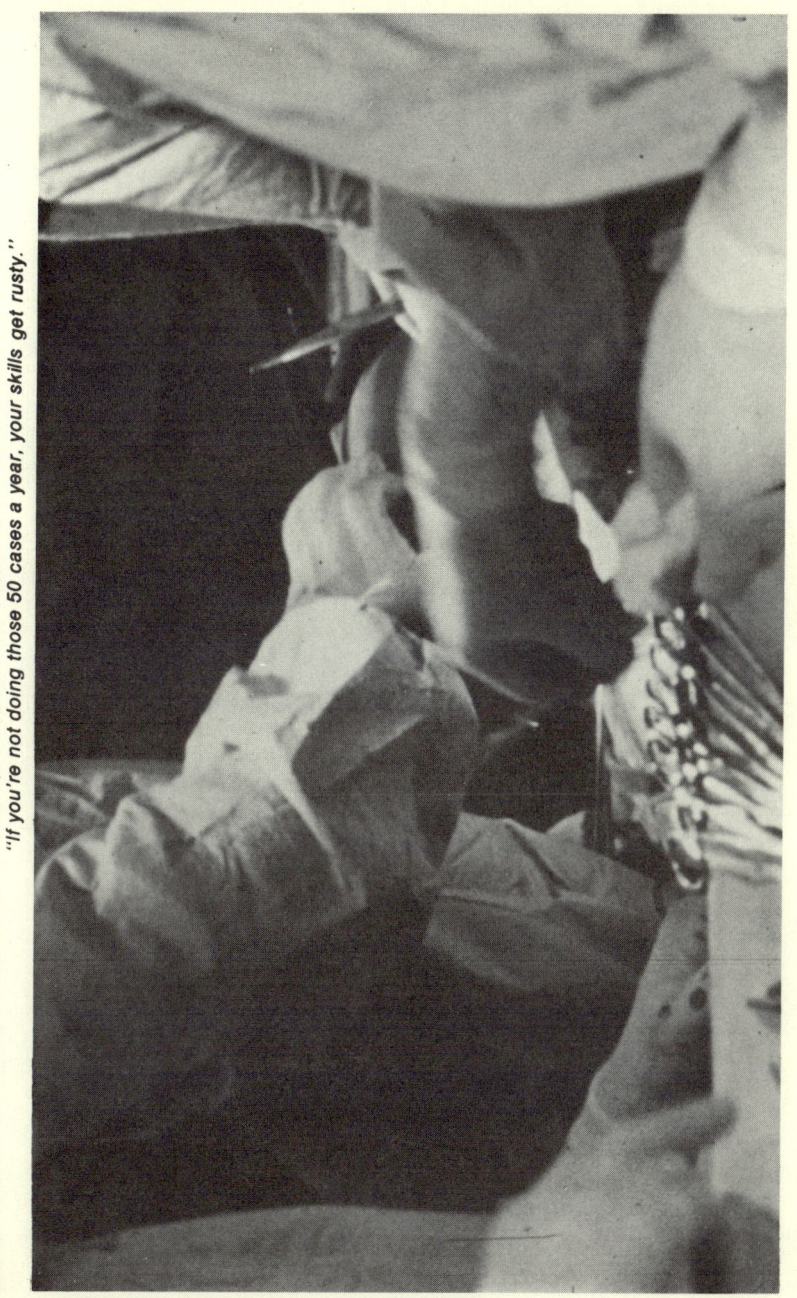

"If you're not doing those 50 cases a year, your skills get rusty."

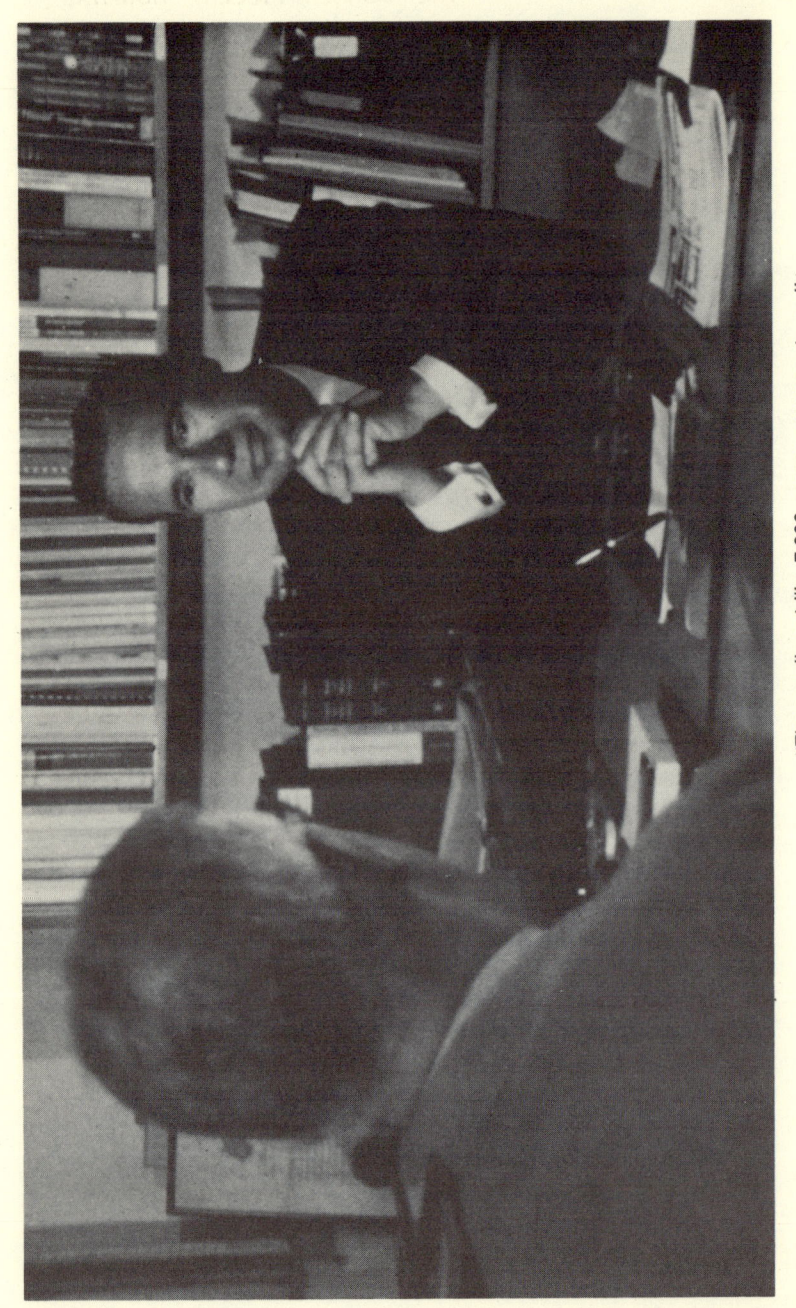

"They really act like 7,000 corner grocery stores."

dialysis unit, which costs $60,000 a year to maintain, a tumor institute, which cost $2 million to install and more than $1.5 million a year to operate, plus an open-heart surgery unit. And much more!

But investigation also turned up some non-standard answers—like equipment duplicated and under-utilized. Mt. Zion's open-heart surgery unit requires a skilled team of twelve doctors, nurses, and technicians maintained on constant stand-by. To function efficiently, it should be regularly doing at least one operation a week. At Mt. Zion, when we were there, it was averaging two a month. Mt. Zion was not alone.

Some 800 American hospitals maintain open-heart surgery as a high-prestige item. In a third of these hospitals, a year can go by without a single operation being performed. Mark Berke, the director of Mt. Zion, said, with refreshing candor, "If you're not doing those fifty cases a year, your skills get rusty, and there's a question about the patient's benefit. As far as I'm concerned, it means that our program is not really necessary for the good of the community. Our surgeons want it, some of our patients need it, but I would say that this is a perfect example of an expensive service that we should perhaps not be offering."

Mr. Berke was also president of the American Hospital Association, and his indictment was a broad one. "We have some 7,000 hospitals, and they really act like 7,000 corner grocery stores. It's difficult to get corner grocery stores to combine their efforts. It's difficult to get hospitals to combine their efforts."

He cited further examples from his own San Francisco experience of expensive duplication:

In San Francisco, as in other large cities which have seen an exodus of young people to the suburbs, there is a surplus of maternity beds. Hospital administrators negotiated an agreement to combine their facilities into one maternity hospital. The hospital directors agreed; the presidents of the boards of trustees agreed; the chiefs of staffs of the hospitals agreed. But the chief of obstetrical service in one hospital balked, and the project fell through.

Mt. Zion's radiation therapy department for tumor treatment is a facility being needlessly duplicated in hospitals throughout the country. "We have physicists, betatron technicians, radiation therapists—all people in short supply. We made a study with a regional planning body, the Bay Area Health Facilities Planning Association, which concluded that no additional facilities were needed at the present time in radiation therapy. Despite this, one hospital has since added a betatron and another hospital is planning to add a linear accelerator. And a third hospital is planning to introduce a radiation therapy department. These require not only huge investments, but trained people. Otherwise you are putting your patients in real jeopardy. And where are all the trained people to come from to man these unnecessary facilities?"

Mr. Berke had a climatic statement when I asked him what the savings would be if America's hospitals were rationally organized, duplication eliminated, and resources properly harnessed for the goal of quality care, efficiently delivered. He thought long before replying:

"If you organized in a total way, with total integration of services, personnel, physicians, and everything else, all designed to provide medical care of the highest quality at the lowest possible price and if you did it within the context of a planned organization for the community, then we would probably find that we have an excess of medical-care beds in the United States. We could reduce them instead of adding to them, assuming an adequate supply of extended-care facilities and nursing-home beds. If we did that, I would guess that we could reduce the national medical bill by twenty per cent. And the patient now paying $117 a day might be paying $100—perhaps even as low as $90. On a national scale that would save billions of dollars."

What is this "total integration" of hospitals that could save billions, and why isn't it happening? These are some of the reforms generally recognized as needed—and being resisted:

1. Area-wide Planning—A community can no longer afford the luxury of hospitals duplicating and under-utilizing expen-

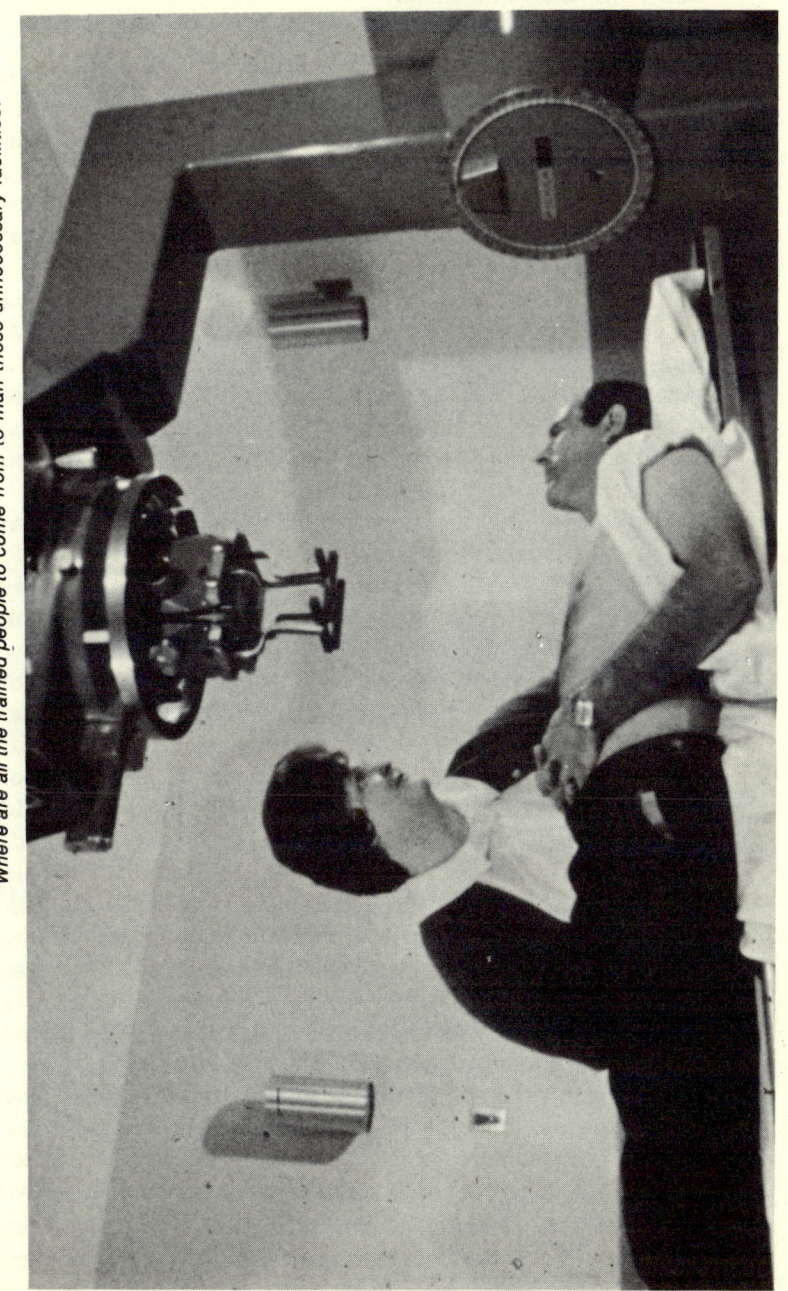

"Where are all the trained people to come from to man these unnecessary facilities?"

sive facilities. Hospitals must be fitted into a central plan which will insure maximum use of facilities.

Walter McNerney, president of the Blue Cross Association, told us, "I think that we should support area-wide planning more energetically than we have. And beyond that, franchisement. That is to say that a hospital cannot start or expand unless its plan has been approved by some authority. For example, banking has it. It is overdue in the health field. ... After all there are many institutions where one manager could run three hospitals better than they are run separately. Laundry, laboratory, and many other facilities could be joined."

But there is not yet enough pressure for such planning. Marke Berke said, "The amount of money that has been poured into hospitals because of government health programs has made such great demands that hospitals which might otherwise have closed down or been absorbed by other institutions, are finding it possible to continue their operations. ... I think that we are going to face the need for some controls. My hope is that it will not be the type of control that would stultify the development of hospitals. But I think that we need controls to make sure that no hospital in any community expands or develops new services unless they meet the needs of the community."

2. Integrating the Doctors—An increasing number of experts recognize the need for what Dr. John Knowles, director of Massachusetts General Hospital, calls "institution-oriented care." That is care built around the hospital rather than around the doctor, who uses the institution as a virtuoso pianist uses a concert hall.

But doctors are scarce and can generally set their terms. The result—operating rooms and facilities that stand idle over weekends, if surgeons do not care to work weekends, and duplication of equipment for the doctor's convenience.

Mr. Berke put it this way, "Some of our unnecessary facilities are maintained because the physicians want them. The role of the institution today is to facilitate the services of the physician. It is inefficient, from his point of view, to have to transfer a patient to another hospital even if he has privileges at that hospital. Often he does not have privileges at the other hospital, so he has to transfer his patient to another physician. He obviously prefers to have all his patients in a single institution with all the services available to him. But this costs the community a great deal of money, and somehow we have to break these patterns down.

"Doctors have to be pulled more closely into hospital operations and have to be involved with the hospital. Doctors today are responsible for more than ninety percent of the costs incurred by the hospital because they admit the patients, they prescribe for the patients, they discharge the patients. They have a great deal of authority over what happens in the hospital with virtually no responsibility for what the hospital has to do to meet his needs."

Dr. George Melcher, president of Group Health Insurance of New York, also urged more doctor involvement with the hospital, but with a greater voice in the running of the institution. "I think," he told us, "that doctors as a group have abdicated their responsibility in relation to in-hospital care. The doctor has little or no opportunity to exert any influence in the hospital as it relates to the services that many of the ancillary personnel perform. And yet these people very much affect the patient's well-being, the time the patient spends in the hospital, and even the outcome of the service rendered."

It is doctors who make the basic decisions about who goes to the hospital and who gets operated on. And Dr. Charles Lewis, of Harvard's Center for Community Health, conducted a study that turned up an amazing fact—that the need for treatment mysteriously seems to rise to meet available capacity. He put it to us this way:

"Parkinson's Law applies in the medical-care system as it now exists. The number of beds available in a community determines the extent of hospitalization. The number of surgeons available determines the frequency of operations performed. The amount of money available for insurance coverage determines the amount of money spent for medical care."

Dr. GEORGE W. MELCHER
PRES. GRP. HEALTH INS.

"Doctors as a group have abdicated their responsibility...."

Rashi Fein, a Ph.D. who is professor of Economics of Medicine at Harvard University Medical School, summed up the problem of the over-utilized hospital and the over-utilizing physician:

"There are a lot of people in hospitals who don't have to be there. You and I don't make those decisions. These are decisions made by physicians. Most of the health dollar is spent as a result of physicians' decisions. You don't walk into a hospital and say, 'I want a bed!' The doctor does that. The question then becomes—are doctors utilizing our hospitals correctly? And I think most observers would say, no, they are not. There is an incentive to put the patient into the hospital. You go into the physician's office and he says, 'You need $200 worth of diagnostic tests, X-rays, etc. Do you want to have them in my office, or do you want to go into the hospital, where you are covered by your health insurance policy?' You're going to go into the hospital! And the physician himself might prefer to have you in the hospital where he can see you on his rounds every day instead of having to pay a visit to your home.

"In this field, in contrast with other, the consumer is not the critical decision-maker. It is the physician. It is his behavior we have to change."

3. Treating Patients Outside the Hospital. As Dr. Fein suggested, there is much that can be more economically and more efficiently done for the patient outside the hospital. Dr. George Melcher, president of Group Health Insurance of New York, told us, "The patient is admitted to the hospital to have many diagnostic studies made that could have been done on an ambulatory basis. This area alone could probably save anywhere from ten to fifteen percent in hospital costs."

But there is much more that can be done outside the hospital walls. In Boston, for example, Massachusetts General Hospital has set up a neighborhood clinic in Charlestown and has treated 5,000 out of the community's 16,000 inhabitants. It has taken over the school health system to improve the examination and treatment of children. Dr. John Knowles, the managing director, says:

"The benefit-to-cost ratio is highest when you extend service to communities which are easily accessible, which practice health education for the people so that they will know more about how to get into the system. We can make better use of scarce manpower. We can treat the undiagnosed case of gonorrhea in the community for $10 instead of spending $4,000 in the hospital six months later when it spreads through the blood-stream into the joints and heart-valves. . . .

"Many hospitals have neglected the development of ambulatory services which can be their window to the community. They can extend their services, keep people on an ambulatory basis, detect disease in its incipiency, prevent disease, rehabilitate disease. I think that hospitals have, in most instances, fulfilled their acutely curative, highly technical, highly costly service very well. But in their rush to acquire more knowledge and carry out this high-cost curative care, they have neglected the extension of their services.

"We know that if we make health services easily accessible to people in the suburbs, as well as to the poor people in the inner city, we can cut their level of hospital admission by as much as eighty percent. And that is the way to save money—to keep those people out of the hospital who shouldn't be there, to treat their disease early so that they don't have to be admitted."

An echo of Dr. Knowles' plea came later in a report of a Federal task force to Elliot Richardson, secretary of HEW. It said, "Priorities should be given to development of organized primary health-care services, especially in neighborhoods with a high proportion of low-income persons, to development of services and resources which can serve as alternatives to hospital care. . . . "

But recommendations like this run up against resistance— resistance compounded of hospitals' attachment to prestige and doctors' attachment to their convenience. We have focused on the hospital because it is the most visible aspect of the health crisis. It accounts for more than a third—$22 billion of the $63 billion health bill. In the past eighteen years, public use of hospitals—measured in days of hospital care—has

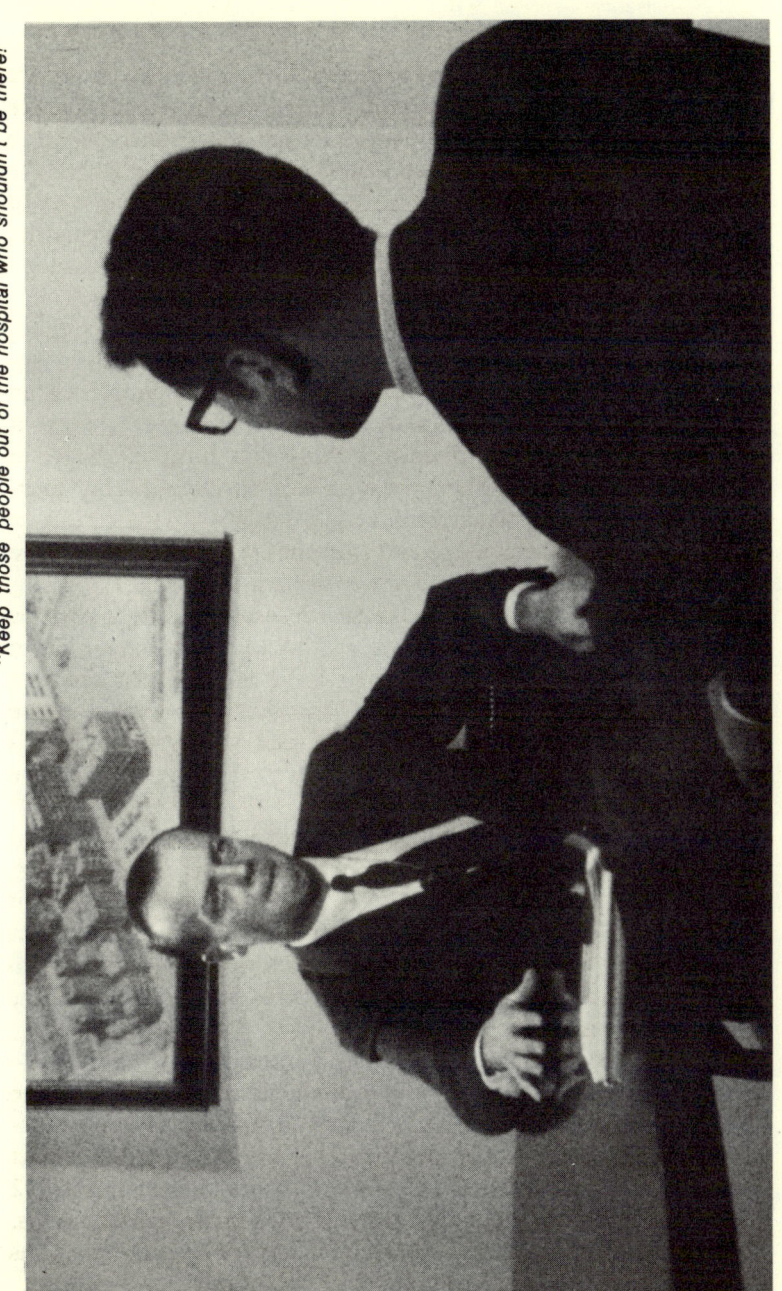

"Keep those people out of the hospital who shouldn't be there!"

increased sixty-nine percent. The American public is now using more than one hospital day per person per year.

The hospital, unlike the disappearing corner grocery-store, still thrives because it is not subject to the control of a free market—and there is as yet no other form of effective control. Much the same can be said for the doctor.

CHAPTER IV
THE "PUSHCART PEDDLER" DOCTOR

DON'T GET SICK IN AMERICA

"The pushcart peddler doctor," said Dr. Rashi Fein, "is the single practitioner making a lot of little decisions. And as long as we have that system, we will have problems."

The term is used because, like the man with his street-corner stand, the physician sells treatment piece by piece. In medicine it is called "fee-for-service," and it is a principle long held sacred by organized medicine.

But the pushcart peddler would envy the doctor's relative immunity to comparison shopping. You must rely on him to decide what item you need and what it will cost. If he doesn't have it in his limited stock, you must then rely on him to refer you to another peddler—the specialist, the surgeon, the radiologist, the pathologist.

Each service has to be separately paid for, each may involve travel and waiting. And, along the way, some of the tests may be repeated, some of the services duplicated.

You have no effective way of checking on the quality of what the solo doctor is selling you. Most doctors are good, but not all. Medicine is a little finicky about self-policing, and only a handful of licenses are revoked a year. Dr. John Knowles, of Massachusetts General Hospital, says, "The marginal practitioner today can sometimes make three times what the best practitioner makes."

Furthermore even the most conscientious men, when in solo practice, find it hard to take time off to keep up with the latest advances in medical science. Dr. Charles Lewis of Harvard told me, "The useful half-life of information now is three to four years. How does a physician in private practice, on a fee-for-service basis, stay current? He must define his own needs, take time off, close the office, lose income, and go off to study."

Many doctors worry about these things, but they do not worry as much as the patients do. In 1968, the National Advisory Commission on Health Manpower reported to President Johnson three danger signals pointing to oncoming crisis—long delays in getting appointments with doctors for routine care, hurried and impersonal attention, and difficulty in reaching doctors nights and weekends. Since then matters

THE "PUSHCART PEDDLER" DOCTOR

have become not better but worse. The doctor feels unfairly criticized. He is working as hard as he can to keep up with growing demands for his services. This year 313,000 doctors are seeing patients about 900 million times outside the hospital—mostly in the doctor's office, of course, seldom do they see patients at home any more.

The answer, some say, is more doctors. There certainly do not seem to be enough to go around. While there are 151 practicing physicians per 10,000 Americans—ten more than in 1950—there are fewer available for the family. More than half the doctors now are specialists. So, for family care there is one per 2,000 people. In the 1930s there were three per 2,000.

And that doesn't begin to describe the problem in areas of doctor scarcity. In some poorer sections of Appalachia, there is one doctor per 7,000 inhabitants. Within one city, Chicago, there are 1.26 physicians per thousand in non-poor areas, but only .62 per thousand, or about half, in the impoverished sections. And two-thirds of America's doctors serve the better-off half of the population.

So, more doctors! In the light of the current shortage, with more than enough business to go around, the organized ranks of physicians are no longer discouraging medical schools from opening their doors to more students, Dr. Gerald Dorman, president of the American Medical Association, told me, "We are expanding as rapidly as we can the number of medical schools, the number of people in medical school, and we are enlarging the number graduating all the time. But the public demand for health is increasing so rapidly that we are not keeping up with the demand."

The plan is to increase the number of medical students by one-quarter to one-half by 1975. But it is estimated that the number would have to double by that time to bring any substantial improvement in the doctor-patient ratio. In any event, it would be a long time before the effect would be seen because it takes a minimum of twelve years to turn a student into a practicing doctor. And, between specialization and the lure of research, only about two percent of the current crop of medical school graduates go into general practice.

Furthermore, current Government budget-slashing in health-care programs threatens some medical schools with curtailment, if not closing. There is some doubt whether even the current modest goals for expanding the ranks of doctors can be attained. Dr. Robert Marston, director of the National Institutes of Health, says there is a problem of rescuing medical schools in danger of going broke. Dr. Roger Egeberg, Assistant Secretary for Health, has told me of trying to see President Nixon to discuss his need for $300 million to help meet the critical shortage of doctors and nurses, only to be short-stopped by Presidential Assistant John Ehrlichman saying that for any discussion of money, another meeting would have to be arranged with the Budget Director present—a meeting that, months later, had yet to be held.

So, an adequate supply of doctors is not likely to appear in the near future. And, even if it did, it would not answer the basic problem of the inefficiency of the "pushcart peddler" system.

The inefficiency has far-reaching effects. Although the average American is spending more than twice as much for health care as he was ten years ago—$270 a person, $14 billion for the nation, representing a growing slice of the Gross National Product—that expenditure is not reflected in gains in the nation's health.

The national death rate, after some spectacular improvements in the postwar period, has held fairly steady since 1950. In some critical areas, the United States appears to be losing ground in comparison with other western countries. The United States has dropped from first to seventh among advanced industrial countries in percentage of mothers who survive childbirth. It is thirteenth in infant mortality, eighteenth in life expectancy for males, and eleventh for females.

Organized medicine correctly declines to accept full responsibility for these statistics, saying they also reflect conditions of poverty, slums, racial problems, and pollution. The doctor, says organized medicine, is doing the best he can. But that should be read as, "the best he can under the present system."

For it is a system characterized by emphasis on acute care over early detection and prevention, a system that presents barriers to getting care when it is needed and when it can be most effective.

"We are perfectly willing," says Dr. Harry Becker of the Albert Einstein College of Medicine, "to spend $5,000 or more taking care of the end result of an illness, like a colon resection on a seventy-year-old person. But we are not willing to spend the same kinds of dollars to catch disease early. And that's a haphazard, upside-down, health-care industry!"

The doctor is a scarce asset, much of whose time today is being wasted doing things that others could do. Dr. Fein cited an example:

"A man goes to medical school, learns how to treat sick children, sets up a practice and spends most of his time treating well babies. Able pediatricians say that eighty percent of the things that a pediatrician does could be done by a well-trained person working under his supervision. Now, we ought to have more people to help the physician so that this very expensive resource would spend his time doing things that only he can do, and not spend his time doing things that other people could do."

But the doctor, basically uncompetitive, does not do what competitive industries do—get management experts to analyze their inefficiencies. There are promising, but small, programs for training assistant doctors—para-medical aides, community health service officers, family health workers. Washington State and Duke Universities have programs for training ex-medical corpsmen returned from Viet Nam to work as physicians' assistants.

But they are not in wide demand. Various reasons are cited—such as the fear of a malpractice suit if an assistant makes a mistake. Doctors seem keenly conscious of the mistakes that others, though supervised, may make but, apparently, are less concerned about the errors that they, though unsupervised, may make. For, at the heart of the resistance to working in harness is the medical cult of the individual, the fact that many choose this profession as one of the last refuges of untrammeled free enterprise. So there is still strong resistance to working in teams.

Despite demonstrated savings in teamwork medicine (the Committee for National Health Insurance estimates that physicians working in groups, aided by skilled aides could serve twice as many patients as the same number of doctors working alone), the medical establishment still chooses to regard team medicine as providing less service than solo medicine.

Dr. Dorman told us, "You've got to have a personnel manager, you've got to have a business manager, you've got to take care of a lot of things that the doctor himself does not do. In group practice, the tendency is also to cut down the number of working hours. Now, if all doctors went on a forty-hour week, we would need fifty percent more doctors today than we have working, because most of our physicians in private practice are working sixty-five to seventy-five hours a week."

The tendency is still to see an organized team of doctors as no more than the sum of its parts and to ignore, not only the benefits of a more rational division of labor, but also the savings that would come from sharing of labor-saving techniques.

There is growing interest, for example, in multiphasic screening, a series of chemical-electronic tests that provide a profile of clinical information on the patient, saving considerable time for the physician in preliminary examination. But Dr. Dorman, in his interview, reflected the old-time solo practitioner's distrust of such new-fangled gadgets.

"Would you rather talk to me or to a machine?" he asked me. "Some people would rather tell the machine. Some people would rather tell the doctor. The doctor can also tell when you are hedging. . . . You have to remember that a computer can only put out what it already had programmed for it. And the programmers have that famous saying, 'Garbage in, garbage out.'"

Multiphasic screening was never intended to be used without a follow-up check by the doctor. It is being introduced into hospitals and into group-practice clinics. But the solo

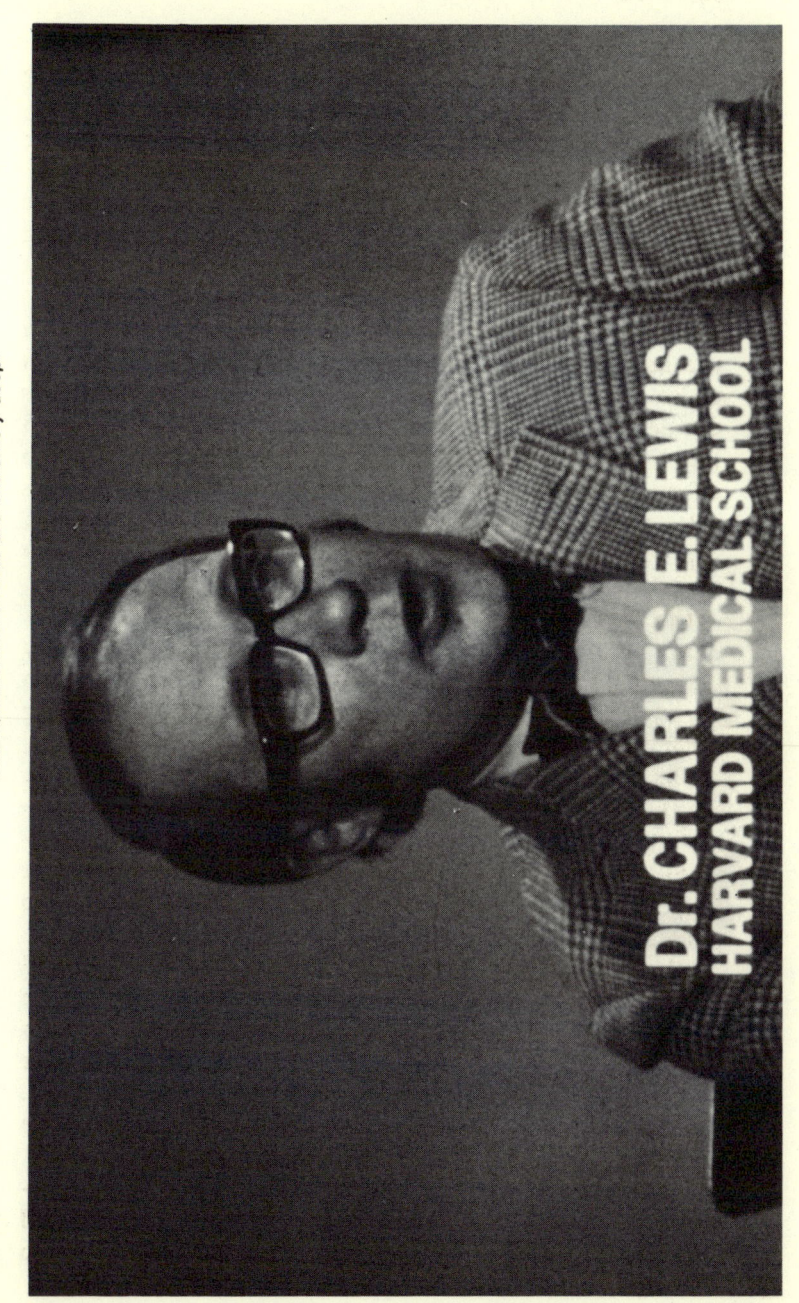

"The establishment roots are extremely deep."

**Dr. CHARLES E. LEWIS
HARVARD MEDICAL SCHOOL**

DON'T GET SICK IN AMERICA

practitioner finds it hard to change, especially when, for so long, he has not found it necessary to change.

"The establishment roots," says Dr. Lewis, "are extremely deep. The problems of organization of medical care can be directly attributed to the manpower problems in medical care. One of the basic problems is the way we select young men for this profession, the way we teach them to think like physicians, to behave like physicians.

"It is not surprising that they reject any sort of group or corporate activity. It takes a long lead time to create a bunch of physicians capable of functioning in groups or in some organized structure."

Some, like Dr. Becker, are pessimistic about reforming today's crop of physicians. He says, "I just don't see the doctors pulling themselves up by their own bootstraps and making creative, innovative changes. They haven't done it in the last quarter century, and the costs are going up. I don't see the American Medical Association out front in talking about the things that we have to do to meet the cost problem, the problem of increasing the supply of people in the health field. I don't see the professional doctors' union, so to speak, in the forefront of change in the direction that we have to go."

Dr. Lewis agrees that change will not come from the medical establishment, but he sees some stirrings among the rank and file, among "the overworked, overcriticized physicians who are basically not part of the political structure of medicine.

"There is," he said, "a silent majority of practitioners, concerned both about the quality of medical care and their own futures. They do not entirely share the feeling that because there is so much money available, there is no reason to change the current system.

"The physician who has functioned in the same way for twenty years is, quite naturally, resistant to change. But some are beginning to perceive advantages in an organization that helps them to define their own shortcomings, helps cover their patients when they are gone, and supports them with income while they are updating their skills."

Even American Medical Association's Dr. Dorman grud-

"We can't wipe out what we're doing now..."

**Dr. GERALD D. DORMAN
PRES. AMER. MEDICAL ASSN.**

gingly concedes that change is coming. "We can't wipe out what we're doing now and suddenly put an entirely new system together. We will develop towards a different system, yes. This I believe. But I don't think that we need—and it would be a catastrophe to have—what's going on now wiped out and an entirely new system put in suddenly."

There seems little danger that the overtaxed, inefficient solo doctor, selling his scarce and intangible wares, will be wiped out overnight. But the pressure is on, not so much from the frustrated but unorganized patient as from the inflation-pinched, large-scale financers of health care.

The insurance companies, said Dr. George Melcher, president of Group Health Insurance of New York, are no longer willing to serve as "simple conduits for money." They are overcoming their long-standing reluctance to get into "delicate areas of patient care."

"The time is just about here," said Dr. Melcher, "when 300,000 physicians are not going to be in a position to tell 200 million people how they're going to get their health care."

CHAPTER V
HEALTH INSURANCE:
THE SHRINKING SECURITY BLANKET

Our novelty wholesaler in San Francisco, Alex Freedman, was hit with the cost of his thousand-dollar hernia operation because he had no health insurance. But fifteen percent of the population, some 30 million Americans, are in his position—most of them because they can't afford it, some of them because they are self-employed and haven't gotten around to taking out personal or family policies. With insurance coverage, he would not have had anything to worry about. Or would he?

Consider George Mastropino, a $5,000-a-year employee at General Electric in Watertown, New York, who had health insurance as a company fringe benefit. His three sons were born afflicted with hemophilia, a hereditary bleeding disorder, which required repeated hospitalization.

Before a Congressional investigation, led by Senator Philip Hart, Mr. Mastropino testified that his insurance had been a godsend—up to a point. It paid $35,000 of the first $53,000 in bills before it was exhausted. Then debts started piling up, bringing judgments and garnishments against his pay. Eventually, with the bad name he got and with loss of time from work because of his sick children, he lost his job. And then things started getting worse.

"I was forced to declare bankruptcy. I had my electricity shut off, my car repossessed. I was not able to obtain credit from anyone. . . . My wife was on the verge of a nervous breakdown." His health insurance, in the end, had covered only a fraction of the $125,000 in medical bills extending over a fifteen-year period.

Or, take the case of Abe Yellowitz, a liquor store manager of Bethesda, Maryland, another witness before Senator Hart's committee. His kidney ailment required an expensive series of procedures, culminating in a kidney transplant. His subscription to Group Hospitalization, Inc., the Washington, D.C., affiliate of Blue Cross, helped considerably—far from completely. Of the first $53,000 in bills, he was left to pay $11,000. And then it developed, as he testified, that "I owed the hospital another $12,500, for which I am now being billed and sued."

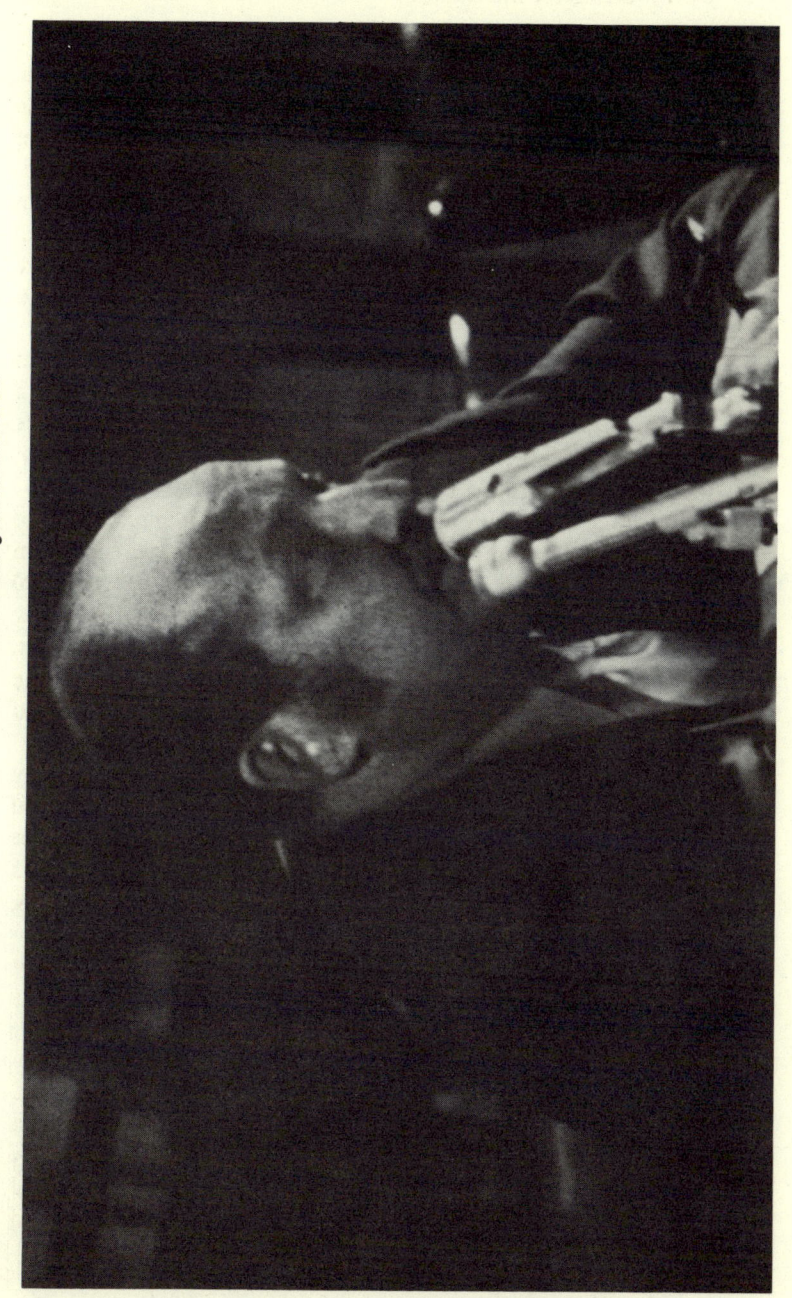

"I am now being billed and sued."

No all-inclusive pass.

HEALTH INSURANCE: THE SHRINKING SECURITY BLANKET

We sat through these hearings as Congress awoke to what many a subscriber had discovered, with dismay, when medical disaster struck—that his insurance was no sure armor against financial peril. In fact, it turns out insurance pays only thirty-six percent of the average cost of sickness. It is best on hospital bills, where it pays an average of seventy-four percent, weaker on doctors' bills, where it pays only thirty-eight percent, and weakest of all on those nagging other costs like drugs and private nursing, where it pays only four percent.

For 170 million Americans who cherish that little insurance card as an admission ticket to the halls of healing, the vast majority find, when they present it at the gate, that it is far from being an all-inclusive pass. More than 60 million have hospital coverage that does not include medical expenses in the hospital. More than 100 million are not covered for treatment in the doctor's office. And then there are "deductibles," the part the patient pays himself, and "co-insurance," the patient's share of payments in some policies.

What has made Americans suddenly aware of their shrinking security blanket is the chill blowing through the widening gap. As insurance companies find themselves no longer able to make ends meet, they have only two possible answers—reduce the benefits or raise the premiums. And their response has been a mixture of the two, plus some changes in the rules of the game. For example, there is less "community rating," where rates are based on spreading the risk among large groups, and more "experience rating," where smaller low-risk groups can pay lower premiums, shunting the high-risk unfortunates off to higher premiums—or insurance oblivion.

For the non-profit Blue Cross-Blue Shield, whose seventy-eight affiliates serve 68 million Americans, some of the recent rate increases have run like this: fifty-six percent for "community-rated" subscribers in New Jersey, fifty-one percent for group members in Connecticut, forty-three percent for "community-rated" subscribers in New York City. And there is apparently more to come. A Federal study has warned that premiums may double in the next five years. A family now paying $469 for a comprehensive Blue Cross-Blue Shield plan may then be paying $907.

The Blue Cross Association had a nationwide survey taken to find out how people were reacting to all this. It expected to find worry among the poor. What it did not expect to find was the extent of worry among the middle-class. The report said that "the economic apprehensions over health are deep and abiding," that "the American people are far from convinced that the economics of health in the United States have been solved," that "most people believe the financial pinch of illness has grown rather than diminished, despite the extended coverage and increased efficiency of medical care." Both poor and non-poor have learned, the survey said, that "many additional expenses are incurred even when supposedly 'covered,'" and subscribers were "shocked" at the amount of money they had to pay for hospital care.

The survey report concluded with a statement that sent up an alarm signal, "This overexpectation . . . of what both insurance and free care will yield to the patient exacerbates the very real feeling that health costs have soared beyond what most Americans feel they can afford. . . . The entire picture is one of on-going worry without any apparent solution as the system is now constituted."

What that means is that the thirty million uninsured—mainly the poor—are being joined in their sense of health insecurity by some of the millions who consider themselves middle-class, and now feel that they are being priced out of the health market. Until recently, ninety-two percent of families with incomes over $10,000 a year had some form of health insurance. Many are finding that their insurance is not adequate, and, at the lower end of the income scale, there soon may be many who cannot afford to pay the high premiums.

This represents a crisis for the $14 billion health insurance industry—the Blue Cross-Blue Shield network, and the 1,500 commercial and private plans that make up a bewildering patchwork of arrangements and benefits. More important, it represents a crisis for the nation, which had come to count on voluntary insurance as the answer to America's health needs.

It is a crisis of special proportions for American business and the American wage-earner. Two-thirds of all Americans who have health insurance are covered by group policies provided at the family head's place of work. Voluntary insurance (some date its inception back to 1847 when a Boston company started providing protection for medical costs and some to the depression days of the 1930s when a group of Dallas school teachers banded together to prepay their care at Baylor Hospital) is really, on its present scale, a product of the era of collective bargaining after World War II. A stimulus was provided by President Harry Truman's proposal for compulsory national health insurance, which produced some nervous shudders. But the big lift came when the trade unions, inhibited in pay demands by inflation controls, began bargaining for "fringe benefits," shifting the burden of health costs to the American employer. American business today is among the loudest who make the groans over the inflation of health costs.

Where did voluntary insurance go wrong? Basically, in turning itself into a golden horn of plenty for hospitals and doctors without strictly controlling the costs, in tipping the American health system towards expensive hospital care instead of preventive and early-illness care, and in pushing the health system to respond more to what is insured than what is needed.

One irony is that insurance helped to push up the hospitals' costs, and in turn, insurance has now become a victim. How this happened was described for us by Dr. Jerome Pollack, associate dean of the Harvard University Medical School, who directed a study in New York State for Governor Rockefeller:

"Very early, when Blue Cross started, it was recognized that cost-plus financing would become very dangerous, that it would remove incentives for economical operation of the hospital. And this, in effect, has happened. Some hospital administrators said that incentives were arrayed on the side

JEROME POLLACK
EXEC. DIR. HARVARD COMMUNITY HEALTH PLAN

"... an open inducement to spend more."

of expenditure. Those who had been economical in previous years found that this worked to their detriment. So, by and large, cost-plus financing has been harmful. A hospital can spend almost all the money it gets. There are so many unmet needs that the method of reimbursement is now seriously deficient. It is an open inducement to spend more.

"We found expenses being charged to the buyers of health insurance which were really incurred in serving the entire community, and not the patients—the cost of education, the cost of stand-by services—and we recommended that these expenses should be charged against the community, and not the patients."

No one knows this better than those who run the hospitals. Mark Berke told us, "Unfortunately the insurance industry, including the Blue Cross and Blue Shield plans, have placed a premium on coming to the hospital. In a way we have oversold hospitals in the United States. We have made them the center of acute care. This has been a good thing in terms of medical care, but the evils are now coming to light."

Doctors' fees have also been affected, as Dr. Rashi Fein described:

"When we have Blue Cross-Blue Shield or commercial health insurance coverage, we know what happens when we go to the physician. He used to charge a certain amount for a procedure. Now he says, 'Do you have insurance?' And when we get the claim from the insurance company, which we don't have to pay, we find that the doctor is charging the company more than he used to charge us. Why? Because we are not concerned, because we don't think the premium is really going to go up very much just because he charged a little more for our procedure. We forget that when all physicians do it, it is bound to have an effect on the premium.

"The physician, when dealing with you or me, may behave very differently than he does when he deals with a post office address—with the thing called an insurance company. The company is something he doesn't meet across the table, doesn't pat on the back and say, 'Take two aspirins and get into bed.' So, there is a behavior pattern involved here. The more impersonal the mechanism, the easier it is to inflate the fee. The company doesn't adequately police it, and things skyrocket. We have, on occasion, seen this happen with automobile insurance. And we have seen it happen with health insurance."

Health insurance has shown other flaws, such as its high overhead in individual policies, which represent more than a fifth of its business. In this area more than forty-six percent of premiums goes not for health benefits but for other expenses. In group policies overhead averages six percent. The more serious indictment, however, is not how insurance does its own housekeeping but what it has done to distort the structure of American health to a pattern that does not meet American needs. The insurance industry now realizes this, and Mark Berke sees a new wind blowing:

"I think that insurance plans are beginning to change. Certainly, we see signs that the Blue Cross and Blue Shield plans are beginning to change, and we see signs that commercial insurance is now going to try to figure out ways of avoiding the acute hospitalization which is the most costly form of care. Medicare and Medicaid have gone a great way toward developing the out-of-hospital concept. They have done much better than the insurance companies, and I hope that the insurance companies will follow their lead."

The leading voice of non-profit health insurance is Walter McNerney, president of the Blue Cross Association. An extensive interview with him indicated an awareness of where insurance has gone wrong and what Blue Cross is now determined to do about it:

"Blue Cross, because it pays most of the bills in hospitals and allied institutions, reflects the costs of these institutions. The fact that the rates are going up is a perfect reflection of the fact that hospital costs have risen so much. We believe in full protection, and we have paid the price for that....

"It is an extremely difficult task to intervene in professional affairs. But we now have active programs of incentives and controls. We watch the claims to see that they are within

"We have paid the price...."

**WALTER J. McNERNEY
PRES. BLUE CROSS ASSN.**

contract. We sponsor utilization review (doctors judging the need for care at the hospital level). We are supporting area-wide planning. We are in a host of activities. The payoffs are slow. Hospitals are much like universities. It is extremely difficult to manipulate care because there is always the jeopardy that you will, at the same time, manipulate quality. But we are, in fact, quite active around the country.

"The membership on our boards has shifted, over the years, from predominantly provider, or hospital representation, to predominantly public representation. And, in accord with that shift, I think that we are displaying more and more public accountability.

"We have two major concerns. One is to provide discipline—incentive controls—so that the money is well spent. At the same time we have to be concerned that services are available when people need them. So, we must be concerned about building hospitals and, secondly, that they not be overbuilt. When we first started, during the depression, the primary thrust was to build because there was a shortage of facilities that continued through World War II. Now the emphasis is less on supply and more on effective demand—that is, arm's length bargaining.

"We have weapons to resist the pressure of the hospitals. One is the community representation on our boards. Another weapon is money. We are the repository of a great deal of money. And through the conditions under which we expend it, we can obviously exercise control.

"We have been guilty, in the past, of underwriting the risk of serious illness rather than addressing ourselves to comprehensive health care. For too many years, our policies were focused on the hospital, which is the most expensive form of care that we have. Now, however, we do underwrite home-care benefits, extended-care facilities, ambulatory benefits, drugs on an ambulatory basis, and we are getting into areas like dental care. The major problem, in this connection, is that not everybody can afford these benefits. In other words, we are increasing the number of products on the shelf; it's up to the consumer to shop for them.

"We have to do more. Our performance, so far, is spotty. We have to make it more uniform in terms of the amount of effort we make. We have to get into other areas. For example, I think that the way we pay hospitals has to be changed. Too much of it is on a cost-plus basis. Once the cost is incurred, it is really too late to do anything about it. So, we are talking more and more about pre-negotiation—offering a rate which the provider of care must live with. Essentially that means that he shares the risk.

"I think that we should throw our weight behind better organization of medical practice. It is absolutely nonsensical that we should not be fully associated with groups of physicians who want to sell their services on a per capita basis. The Blue Cross subscriber should have a choice. If he wants a solo practitioner, fine! But if the physicians want to organize in groups, we should be fully associated with and supportive of that. Potentially there is a lot of productivity in that type of move.

"I think that we can make better use than we have of our computers, and we are beginning to do it. We have now stored in our memory banks all types of information. Why not start to set some parameters and begin to ask some serious questions about variations in utilization that are so far inexplicable so that the hospital and the physician are continually enjoined to be careful about the economy of care, as well as the quality of care?"

Some of the commercial insurance companies are now also, however belatedly, looking for more efficient health systems for their subscribers. "There is now," says Harvard's Dr. Pollack, "a certain ferment, a certain creativeness among voluntary insurers. There is a classic pattern, in other countries, of having voluntary plans precede governmental ones. There is a role for insurance companies in encouraging invention in the way that health services are organized. And if the private carriers are willing to be experimental, this is much to be encouraged."

An alarmed health insurance industry was now ready to apply some of its $14 billion leverage toward controlling costs and, more important, toward prodding the health industry into the twentieth century. It needed the additional leverage of the Federal Government, long inhibited by a potent medical lobby from trespassing on the sacrosanct preserve of ministering to the nation's health.

CHAPTER VI
THE TRAUMA OF MEDICARE AND MEDICAID

In 1965, the Federal Government, after a four-and-half-year donnybrook with organized medicine, took its first plunge into the untried waters of health-care financing for large groups of Americans, and five years later was floundering in desperation. Through Medicare, for the aging, and Medicaid, for the poor, the Government went in to rescue the most vulnerable groups of our population, the ones largely neglected by private insurance. But, with no plan for harnessing the swelling torrent into more coherent health channels, the Government raised the inflation tide to flood level—for itself and for the public—and found itself up to its neck, gasping for breath.

As we turned to our examination of Uncle Sam as a sponsor of health care, we found a sense of spreading consternation among Administration and Congressional policy makers. One Congressional committee after another called hearings and filed reports crying havoc. Few seemed able to discuss the situation without panicky phrases like "crippling inflation" and "threatening breakdown." Officials blinked at projections showing costs zooming off into space. Between 1965 and 1970, Federal spending for medical assistance increased fivefold, and Senator Russell Long, chairman of the Senate Finance Committee, warned of a staggering deficit of $216 billion for Medicare over a period of twenty-five years.

Retreat and abandonment of the aging and the poor were not possible (though some of the newer Republican hands in the Administration raised that possibility at closed-door crisis sessions). To continue simply pumping in ever-increasing amounts of money was not possible either. Like the private insurance industry, the Government manned the dikes with sandbags of higher premiums and lower benefits. It issued stern orders to control the rise in costs. But beyond that the Government began to confront the realization that something more fundamental had to change.

That something was the one thing that Congress, back in the days of innocence in 1965, had crossed its heart and sworn to organized medicine not to change—how health services are delivered to Americans. There are weak grins now when one recalls the free-enterprise safeguard clause that was written into the Medicare law, forbidding the government to "exercise any supervision or control over the practice of medicine or the manner in which medical services are provided."

This clause reflected the spirit of accomodation to organized medicine which resolved the battle that had raged through the Kennedy and early Johnson Administrations. Title XVIII of the Social Security Act, a landmark in social legislation, made about 20 million people over the age of sixty-five the first large group of Americans to be recognized as having an inherent right to health care. But along with the mandatory hospital insurance system, its burden spread by being based on social security payroll taxes, other features were added under pressure from organized medicine—a Medicare optional Part B, to finance physicians' services, and, almost as an afterthought, a Title XIX launching Medicaid as a virtually open-ended commitment to finance services for the poor and the near-poor from general tax money on a generous matching basis with the states. Enshrined in the law were the principles of paying "reasonable costs" rather than fixed prices, to hospitals, and "reasonable" or "customary fees" to physicians. These concessions started a time bomb ticking.

The price of health care, which had been rising at a rate of three percent, suddenly began rising at six percent. What had been intended as a price ceiling had become a price floor.

"With the advent of Medicare and Medicaid," recalls Dr. Rashi Fein, "physicians became price conscious. They were afraid that the Government would eventually have to freeze prices. And, if you're sitting around speculating on whether prices are going to be frozen, you want to get your fees up as high as you can before the freeze comes. Doctors are humane; they are also human. So Medicare and Medicaid contributed to price increases, not because of demand conditions, but because physicians were permitted to charge more. Prices would have gone up somewhat, but they were pushed up further by Medicare and Medicaid."

"In the case of hospitals," said Dr. Fein, "we did have

an increase in demand because of Medicare. The aged population does use hospitals. That's exactly what we wanted, and we anticipated that. But many of our hospitals were operating close to capacity and, with a little more push, they were faced with higher costs. The Federal Government had said, 'We will help you meet your costs.' It did not say, 'We will give you an incentive to try to operate efficiently.' And so hospitals increased their purchases of capital equipment, buying things they had wanted all along but could not afford. Many of these things are good. Many of them are probably unnecessary in every hospital. . . .

"What happened could have been anticipated. Theoretically, better legislation could have been written. But it is questionable whether better legislation could have been enacted in 1965. The American public had to learn that controls and intervention into the system are not just things that economists and some Congressmen like but that they may be necessary. I do not think that lesson would have been learned without undergoing the experience."

The "experience" is higher costs and inadequate care for many. The Federal Government is now spending $19 billion a year on health—more than the whole country spent fifteen years ago. The Government's share of the national health budget rose from twenty-five to thirty-seven percent in three years. Medicare and Medicaid are costing the Federal Treasury $14 billion a year, double the expected figure, and could easily reach $20 billion by 1975. The Senate Finance Committee says, "The Medicare and Medicaid programs are in serious financial trouble."

It isn't only the Government that is in trouble, but the beneficiaries. Premiums rose and benefits were curtailed. For hospital care, Medicare beneficiaries must now pay the first $52 of their bills, instead of $40, as in 1966. And Social Security actuaries say that "deductible" is likely to reach $84 by 1974. The premium for the voluntary medical part of Medicare has jumped from $3 to $5.30 a month—an increase of more than seventy-five percent. And coverage is far from complete. The Government says it is paying forty-five percent

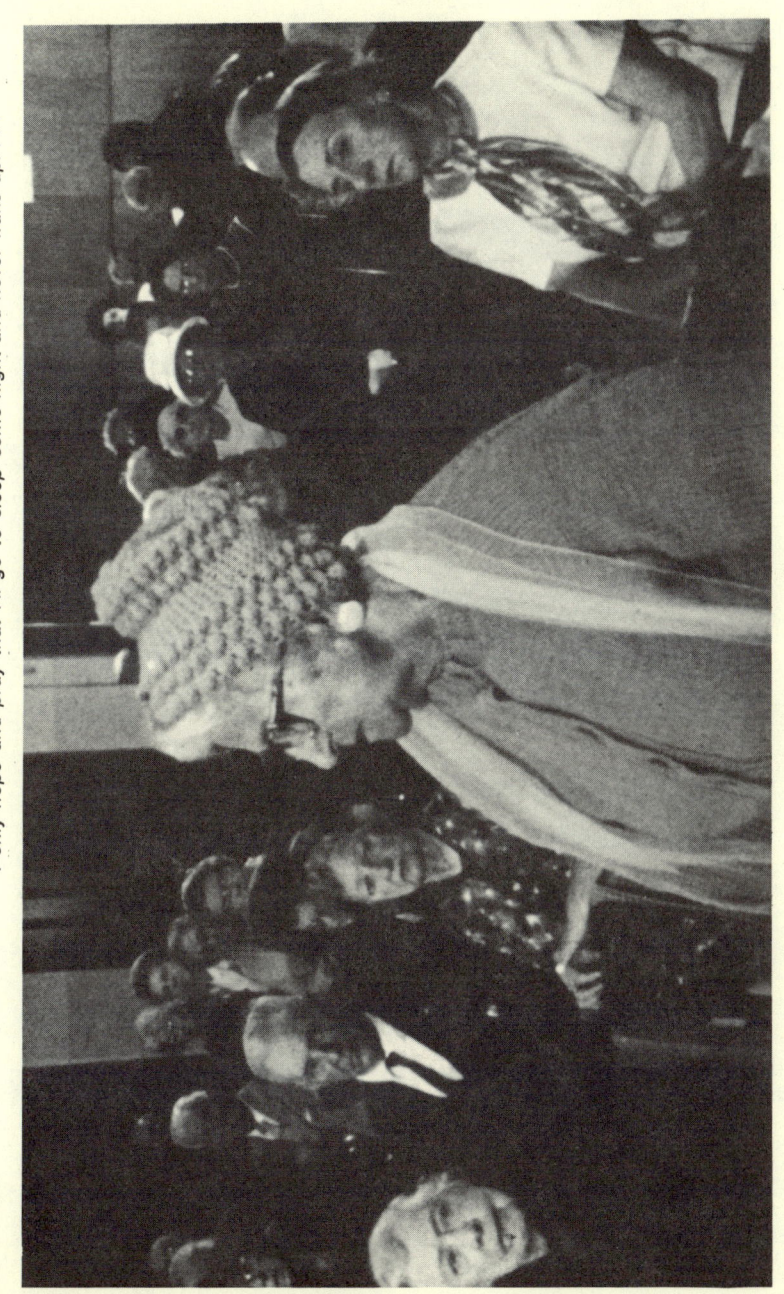

"I only hope and pray that I'll go to sleep some night and never wake up...."

of the health bill of our senior citizens. Outside analysts figure it is actually closer to thirty-five percent. Old people who are billed directly by their doctors often have trouble collecting in full from the insurance companies that serve as intermediaries for the Government.

There is something dry and impersonal about percentages, deductibles, and restrictions. To see how some of our senior citizens are faring under Medicare, we went to St. Petersburg, Florida. We attended a meeting of old folks and heard a torrent of grievances about the ruinous expenses left after Medicare had paid its share, about the high cost of medicine out of the hospital that Medicare does not pay for.

We listened to an old lady say, "I only hope and pray that I'll go to sleep some night and never wake up, if I'm supposed to be sick, because what I hear, all these medical bills and all the doctor bills that people have to pay, and they worry about it. I hope I never have to go through that."

We listened at length to Miss Patricia Bell, a Florida State welfare worker, recounting with passionate indignation the plight of some of her Medicare cases:

"I have one lady, and we can't buy teeth for her. Medicare won't pay for them. So she goes home from the nursing home after being fed on soft foods until she comes up to a certain weight. Once home, she can't eat because she doesn't have any teeth. So she gets sick again and goes back into the nursing home. And this is a cycle that goes on and on. . . .

"There are people who are totally bed-ridden because they can't afford to get glasses. There's no allowance in Medicare for this type of thing. . . .

"I saw a woman today who has crippling arthritis. Her fingers turn up. She's sixty-five years old and can't get out of bed. Medicare won't pay for any kind of nursing care, so she had to apply for old-age assistance to pay a practical nurse to take care of her because she can't do anything for herself. She can feed herself, and that's it. She can't comb her hair. She lies in bed, and she's been lying there for three months. She hasn't been to the doctor for two-and-a-half months because she can't afford to pay him. If she had the

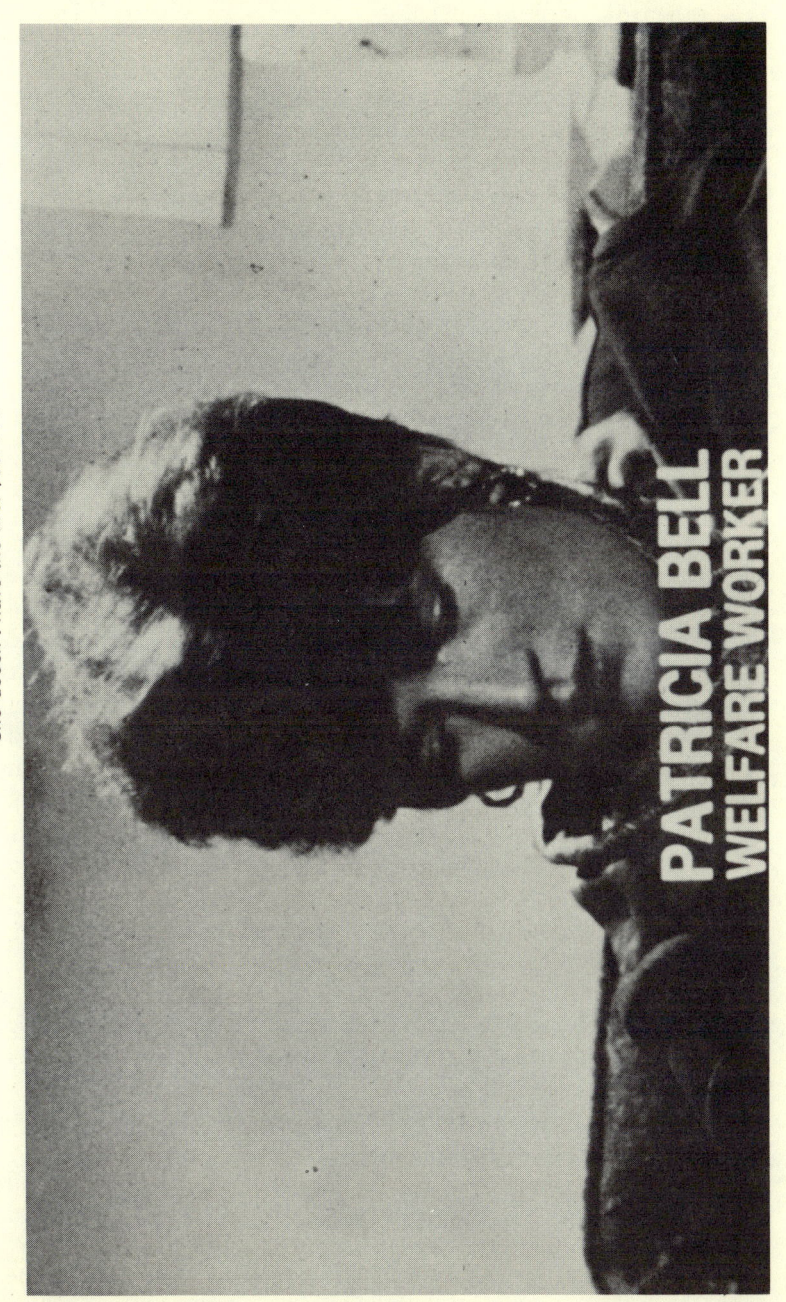

"She doesn't have the first $50. . . ."

**PATRICIA BELL
WELFARE WORKER**

doctor, she might get better. Nobody will ever know because she can't pay the doctor. She doesn't have the first $50. . . .

"I have one lady who was in a nursing home. She should have stayed in a nursing home, but she had to go home because her Medicare ran out. She had no money. She went home to an alcoholic son, who beats her. She can't go back to the nursing home because she can't pay for it. Medicare won't cover it. So she has to stay there and be beaten at eighty-five years of age. . . .

"One man had two-thirds of his stomach removed. The operation was $5,000. Medicare paid all but twenty percent, which left him with $1,000 to pay. Well, his income is a little over $1,000 a year. It will take the rest of his lifetime to pay it."

But at least Medicare has provided substantial help for twenty million elderly Americans and eased the strains on their children. More dismal has been the Medicaid experience. At considerably greater cost per person, it has reached only about 12 million of the poor and near-poor, little more than a quarter of its target population of 40 million and reached them under forty-eight widely varying state programs (Arizona and Alaska have none), through a tangled maze of bureaucracy and eligibility requirements. A Federal task force reported that Medicaid reaches "a minority of the poor and near-poor today, and there is some question of the extent of the need which is met even where they are reached."

How far Medicaid has fallen short of its goals is revealed in facts and in figures like these:

Only twenty-eight states gave Medicaid coverage to people not on welfare, but poor enough to be considered "medically needy."

A third of the states have reduced services and cut recipients off the rolls by tightening eligibility requirements.

The deadline for states to make services available to all those eligible has been postponed from 1975 to 1977—and may be eliminated entirely.

The watchdog staff of the Senate Finance Committee made

an exhaustive study that found several thousand doctors earning more than $25,000 a year—in some cases, more than $100,000—by assembly-line treatment of Medicaid patients. It demanded "prompt action" by organized medicine to monitor the care provided and the fees charged, warning that the alternative would be "control procedures which may be arbitrary, rigid, and insensitive to the legitimate needs of both the patient and his physician." Senator Long spoke of the "grab-bag attitude that has apparently characterized" the Medicare-Medicaid programs.

We asked Dr. Gerald Dorman, president of the American Medical Association, for his views on the escalation of fees.

"There were many times when we used to care for our older patients at a lower fee, or free," said Dr. Dorman. "The Government said that there shall be no more free medicine. Everybody must be paid for it. And we have doctors, not only under Medicare but also in Medicaid, who have made a large income because they are working with the people who are poor, who come under these programs of Government care. We have one doctor out in Oakland, California, for instance, who made over $100,000. That was checked over, and it was found that he had earned it. . . . There's another doctor up in Hartford who made over $25,000, and the Government down in Washington said that anyone over $25,000 should be investigated. He says, 'Let them come in and look at me,' because his practice is in the poor area.

"Now, in the old days before Medicare and Medicaid, these people would have been treated free or for a minimal fee. We've had people up in Harlem who were treated for a fifty cents office fee, which seems incredible. . . . But these things have changed. We want to see the poor treated as anybody else in the country, as private patients, so that they get the best possible care."

Dr. Dorman warned that there could be serious consequences if the Government tried to hold down fee schedules. He said, "Where they have been fixed—in Belgium, in France, in Italy—we have found that after five years, or ten years, the Government tends to say, We fixed your fees. You agreed to them. There they are! We have other priorities—for roads, for education, for work abroad, for trips to the moon. . . . In the long run, if doctors cannot make ends meet, there will be a tendency not to go into medical care."

Dr. Rashi Fein discounted the prospect of a doctors' rebellion against cost controls. "Unhappiness? Yes. Rebellion? I don't know what that would mean here. We admit about fifty percent of the applicants who apply to medical school, and a very high percentage of those rejected are fully capable. Everyone agrees that we could expand medical enrollment. . . . As I meet students today in medical school, I'm convinced that these are highly motivated young men who want to do things in social settings where they feel they are accomplishing things. . . . I'm not saying that they'll feel the same way five years from now. Given the system of medical practice in the United States, many will, in time, be induced to behave as other physicians have. But I don't see a rebellion. . . .

"I think that organized medicine will be taken on. And, as we have seen the problem of establishing civilian control over the military, so we will have to have civilian control over the health sector."

And that is starting to happen! Rebellion or no, the Government has moved to check the rise in its health costs. It has put ceilings on Medicaid payments to physicians and introduced legislation to set controls on increases to doctors that Medicare will recognize. It has asked Congress for authority to negotiate with hospitals in advance on what rates they will charge the Government. And, with one blast, HEW proposed to sweep away the premise on which Medicare and Medicaid started. "Neither the reasonable cost nor the reasonable charge criteria established in the law," it stated, "have provided opportunity for major cost-control efforts. . . . It is now time to make some fundamental changes."

But trying to clamp the lid on the boiler was not redesigning the engine. As long as new money was pumped into an old system, it would tend to produce higher costs rather than more services. Medical Economist Herman Somers of Princeton University summed up the broader problem when he

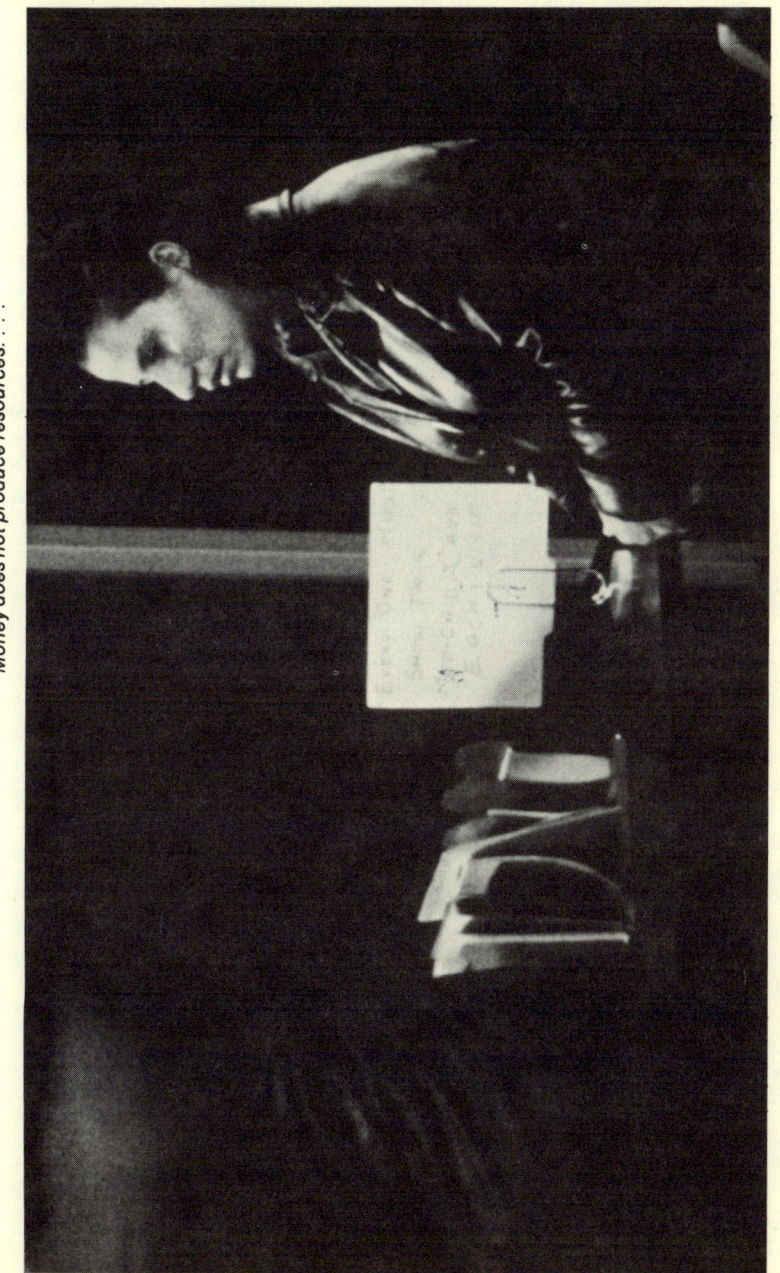

"Money does not produce resources...."

said, "The availability of money does not produce resources where they do not exist. . . . Additional expenditures have not only failed to produce equitable utilization of health care resources by the whole population, but there has been small net gain."

The Federal Task Force on Medicaid, headed by Walter McNerney, reported to HEW Secretary Elliott Richardson that "the Medicaid program, by structure and financing, is deficient, and, in its present form, it is unlikely that the goals of reasonably adequate and uniform coverage and effective controls on costs and quality can be achieved." It asked that Medicaid be converted into a Federal program with a uniform level of benefits—as a first step. Beyond that it looked to "a national policy of financing health care."

Up to its neck now, the Federal Government could not retreat. Its situation was likened by Dr. Rashi Fein to someone standing waist-deep in a cold lake, shivering and wondering whether to get out or start swimming to get warm.

"I don't think the Government has any choice. It is not going to jump out. It responded to the needs of the people, to the social climate of this country. I think it now has to get in all the way. It has to be concerned not only with the financing of medical care, but with the delivery system. It's going to have to take sides."

Now, Walter McNerney said that the 1965 pledge not to intervene in the way medical services are provided "cannot be taken seriously." And attention began turning to what could be done about this amorphous thing called "the delivery system."

CHAPTER VII
"KEEP WELL!"—THE DRIVE FOR HEALTH MAINTENANCE

Invention, daughter of necessity, can remain a neglected child until a father appears to give her name and respectability.

The newest rage of the Government health establishment is something represented by the mysterious abbreviation, "HMO." It stands for Health Maintenance Organization, which is bureaucratese for "Prepaid Group Practice," which is medicalese for a system of paying a fixed annual sum to a group of doctors to keep you well when they can and cure you when they can't.

To hear people talk about it, you would think the idea was born yesterday. Blue Shield in California has come up with a version of it. A catchy folder tells subscribers of "the 'Keep Well' plan you've been waiting for . . . Now for the first time . . . based on a new concept."

Prepaid Group Practice actually started in this country in 1938 when Industrialist Henry J. Kaiser, seeking to lure workers to remote construction sites, offered to look after their health for five cents a day. By 1945, the Kaiser Foundation Health Plan was ready to go public, and today the Kaiser workers are almost lost among the two million subscribers in five states. Kaiser is still expanding at a rate of ten percent a year, and in some areas turns applicants away because it cannot expand fast enough.

It would have spread faster but for the bitter hostility of organized medicine, long wedded to the principles of "solo practice"—the single, free-enterprise virtuoso physician—and "fee-for-service"—separate payment for each separate item of doctor's care. The influence of the medical lobby has helped to write prohibitions or restrictions on Prepaid Group Practice into the statute books of more than half of our states.

Official investigations have given Kaiser high marks for economy and efficiency, for catching illness in early stages, for avoiding illness by timely preventive care, for reducing hospital stays by an average of forty percent, for providing "one-stop shopping service" and for making access to health care easy. Senator Abraham Ribicoff, former Secretary of HEW, listened incredulously in 1968 to testimony that Medi-

"KEEP WELL!"—THE DRIVE FOR HEALTH MAINTENANCE

care beneficiaries enrolled with Kaiser in Oregon were using little more than half the hospital time of the national average Medicare patient. And, because Medicare was paying for hospital days, not for efficiency, Kaiser was, in effect, being penalized for its performance.

We decided to have a long look at the Kaiser operation in California.

Under a typical Kaiser plan, a family of three or more was paying $35.40 a month for hospitalization up to 111 days a year, office treatment at $1 a visit, house calls for $5. This includes all surgery, X-rays, and laboratory tests. In some plans, maternity care is free; in no case is it more than $100.

In the Los Angeles appointment center, the clerks, with their spinning racks of cards, were receiving a thousand calls a day for 250 doctors in ten medical offices. These were, among the 2,000 doctors, combined into partnerships, paid salaries averaging $36,000 a year, plus bonuses when annual costs ran under estimates. The appointment center looked huge and impersonal, but most patients were making appointments with doctors of their choice, doctors they had seen before. In random interviews we tried to learn how subscribers liked the Kaiser system.

A woman: "I have been a member of the plan since 1953. There is nothing else I know of that meets the needs of the middle-class and the working people. Generally, the care is very good, especially if one has a serious illness. Less urgent cases don't always get the best service. They have to wait longer in clinics. But I think this is also true in the private doctor's office today."

Another woman: "Right now my daughter is in for some minor surgery. It won't cost me a dime. The premiums have paid for everything. The care has been excellent. The service is in-and-out. You make an appointment, and the service is right there. I selected a doctor whom I have seen from time to time, and I am quite satisfied."

A man: "I have had four hernia operations. Right now I am here for X-rays. The operation didn't cost me one red

A thousand calls a day. . . .

"KEEP WELL!"—THE DRIVE FOR HEALTH MAINTENANCE

cent, and neither do the X-rays. You get the best care there is. I've had the same doctor all through."

A woman: "I came here two years ago from New York, where I had Blue Cross and Blue Shield. Since we joined Kaiser I can't speak highly enough of them. They've done wonders for my husband. He had a heart attack, and he's been coming here every couple of weeks. They've done a lot for him. They're just fantastic!"

Another woman: "I've had two major operations. Didn't cost a penny. I was in just this last year for a hysterectomy. I had nurses practically around the clock. I mean, they're just in and out, checking on you all the time. It's really something!"

A man: "I had a very much needed operation resulting from a birth defect. My hips had grown shut. I wasn't able to bend. They put a steel ball in each hip—two operations. I was in the hospital sixty-seven days the first time, six weeks the second time. The only thing I had to pay for was my crutches—and for the TV and telephone while I was in the hospital. I know a lot of people have felt that Kaiser is bad because they think the doctors are not good. But I think I had a very good doctor."

Another part of the story is how Kaiser can provide service for an average of twenty-five percent less than equivalent fee-for-service care—by planning for maximum utilization of personnel and facilities. Kaiser does not have expensive prestige installations in every hospital. It has found it cheaper and more efficient to bring a patient to a facility and provide an apartment during treatment. Mrs. Cathlyn Albanese of San Diego told us a typical story:

"About Thanksgiving time I had an operation at the Kaiser Hospital in San Diego and they discovered that I had cancer. They don't have cobalt equipment in the Kaiser Hospital in San Diego but they do have in Los Angeles. I was concerned because I thought it would be very expensive and that I would have to pay for an apartment. They told me that I didn't, that a completely furnished apartment would be provided at no cost. It is a quite large one-bedroom apartment, and

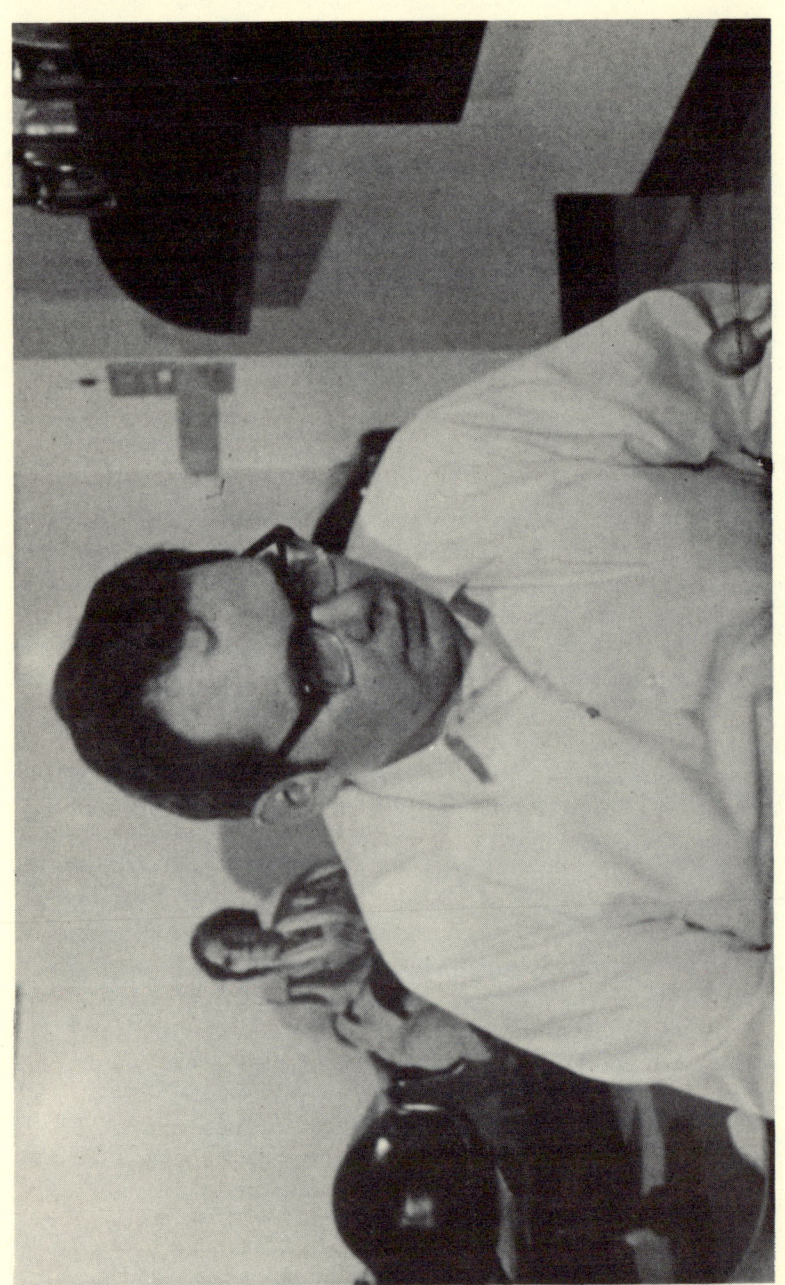

"The only thing I had to pay for was my crutches."

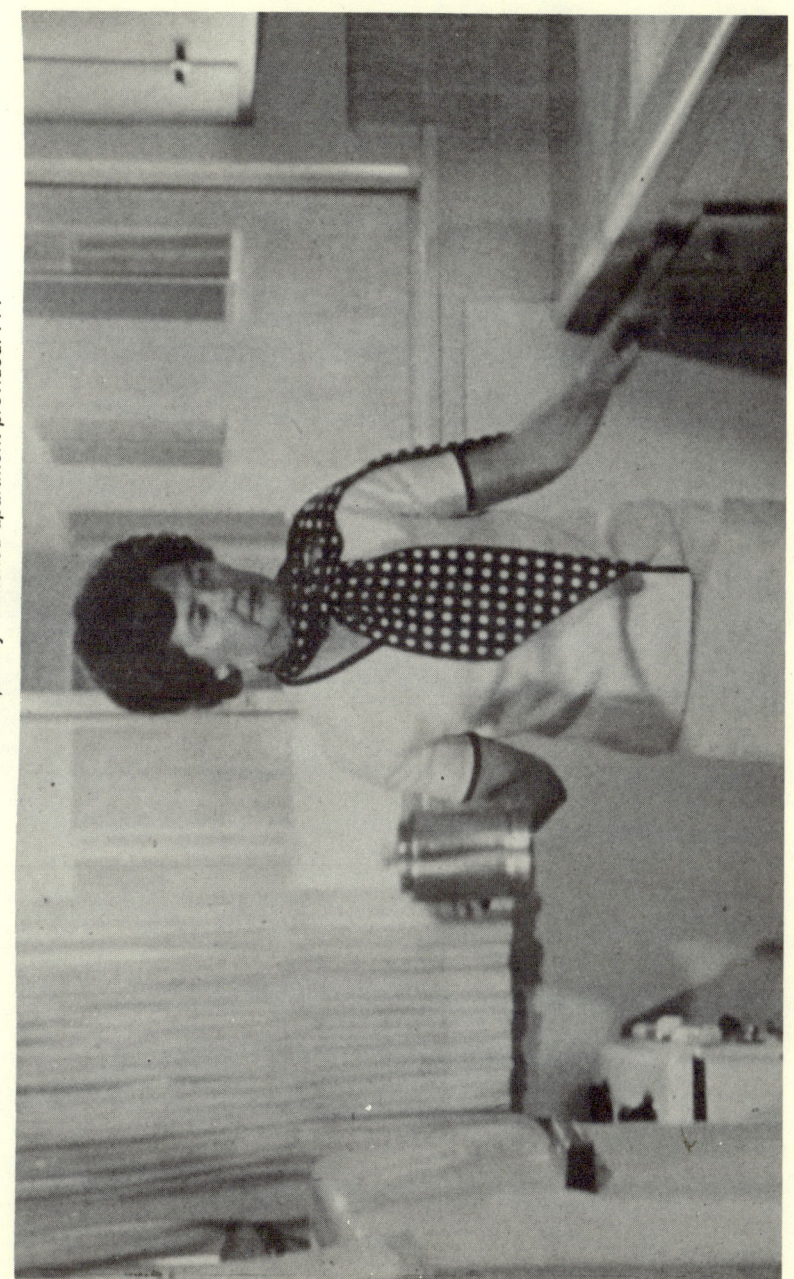

A completely furnished apartment provided....

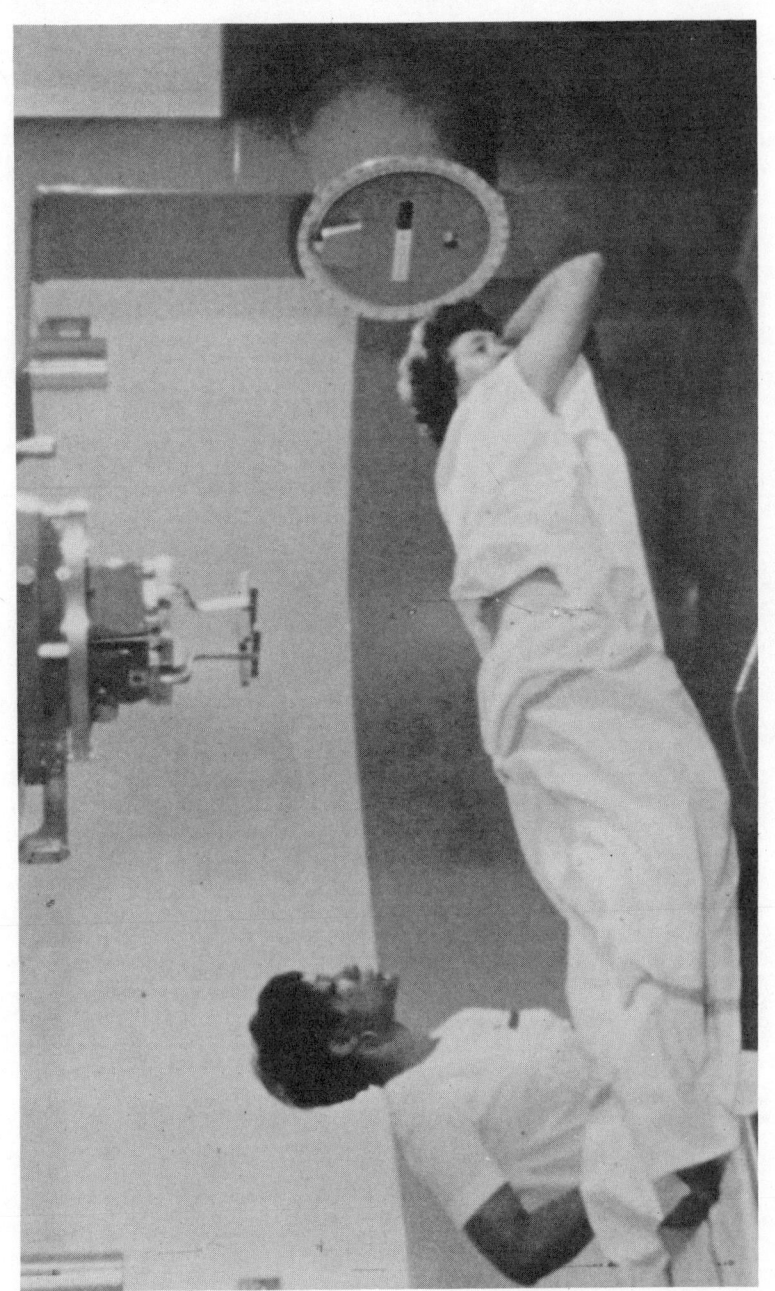

"The cobalt treatment won't cost me anything. . . ."

"KEEP WELL!"—THE DRIVE FOR HEALTH MAINTENANCE

it has maid service. My husband comes up on weekends and takes me home. I'll be here for six to eight weeks—approximately thirty-four treatments. The cobalt treatment won't cost me anything. It's all furnished with the plan."

Because Kaiser makes its money from good health, not illness, there is a strong accent on prevention. Children are brought by their parents periodically to "well baby clinics" to be checked by pediatric nurses—thus freeing doctors to treat sick children.

One of the most frequent criticisms of organized practice is that the doctor becomes a cog in the system and loses his sense of incentive. We interviewed a Kaiser physician, Dr. Paul Roth, internist, who was considered a maverick when he joined Kaiser in 1955. As a partner in the physicians' group, he is paid $38,000 a year and shares in bonuses when annual costs are under estimates. This is Dr. Roth's story:

"I joined because I wanted to be able to practice good medicine, and I wanted to have my family life. I know what my hours are, and I know that when I'm off, I'm off—free to be at home, to leave my home, and leave no telephone number. I know that my patients are being taken care of by fellows who are competent, so that I know that I don't have to worry about them.

"When I first came here, directly from medical school, I felt some criticism from the County Medical Society. There was a lot of talk about whether good medicine would be practiced at Kaiser. There was a lot of difference of opinion. I had some doubts, too. I had to find out for myself.

"I think that I practice as good medicine as I can. I see about eighteen patients a day. In private medicine I'd probably see more and have less help in doing it. Whether I'd make more money in private practice I don't know. I have enough. Overall, I've been content.

"I don't think large group practice is good for everybody. I think it depends on what your goals are, what you want out of life, how well you function in a group setting. I guess we don't get the ego satisfaction of having developed our own practice, with financial reward as a measure for success.

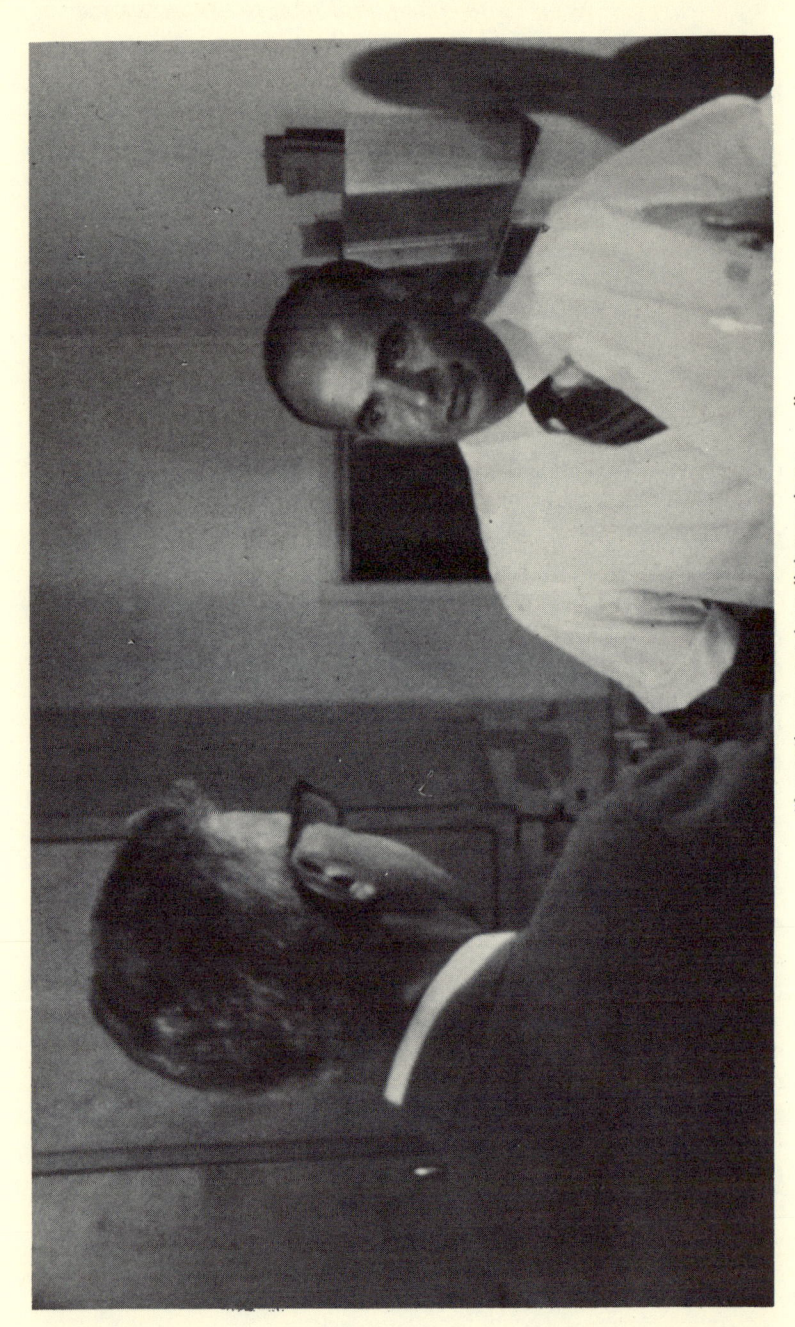

"*I practice as good medicine as I can. . . .*"

"KEEP WELL!"—THE DRIVE FOR HEALTH MAINTENANCE

We also get the feeling of being judged by the other doctors. I guess that there is nothing quite as concrete as having an ever-increasing number of patients, putting an ever-increasing number of dollars down to get your care. Well, I don't need that, but I think a lot of doctors do.

"Also, some doctors would object to having schedules made out for them. They feel that they want to make out their own time schedules. I think that's a little naive. I think that in individual practice, though I've never been in it, your bosses are your patients collectively. You really are not free to take off at the drop of a hat and go sailing. So maybe we lead a more structured life, part of it not under our control, but I don't think doctors have things under their control anyway.

"For the patients, when it comes to the nitty-gritty of how well they will be treated medically, I don't think that this can be beat. At the same time, I think that there are some inconveniences that the patients object to. For example, waiting, especially when they don't have appointments—the so-called emergency patient, who usually is not an emergency, but may think he is. We haven't found a way to beat that yet. Maybe we never will. We used to think that we could educate the patients to call and make appointments so that we wouldn't run into this problem so often. And that we could get them to come more during the day than in the middle of the night."

Prepaid group practice is not utopia. But James P. Vohs, executive vice-president of the Kaiser Health Plan, summarized for us the improvements he believes it has brought about:

"It is easy access to the system and the opportunity for a more coordinated approach to a person's medical management, a continuity of care. The key feature of our approach is the assumption of responsibility to plan and deliver and to organize medical services. No component of our system can afford the luxury of indifference to what is going on in other parts of the system. The physicians' groups, the health plan, and the hospitals function as a coordinated, interdependent enterprise.

"We believe that group practice offers a mechanism to increase the supply of services that a given number of physicians can render. We think that you can influence economy and efficiency if you group physicians together in organized settings and in centralized locations, if you put the physicians' offices in the hospital, thereby reducing the travel time for the physician. He's able to share facilities, equipment, and personnel. And when you do as we have done, and link these inpatient and outpatient facilities in a coordinated manner, you avoid unnecessary duplication of equipment and services. When you collect services that would be low-volume and very expensive—open-heart surgery, deep-radiation therapy, the betatron—into a central medical center, there are economies that result. . . .

"In all of this, we have found no loss in the doctor-patient relationship. We encourage members to select an internist, for example, as the key family physician, and to select a pediatrician. When they require care, they always go back to see those physicians. And there a relationship is built. The economic barrier is removed. We think that there is an opportunity to develop an even warmer, stronger relationship between patient and physician.

"There is no incentive in our program for the physician to follow a course of treatment for the patient other than what his best judgment would dictate to him. He is not influenced by the ability of the patient to pay. Nor does he feel pressured to provide a certain kind of treatment because that's the kind of service that's covered. In our comprehensive program, inpatient and outpatient services are covered.

"I think this should lead to encouragement for more plans of our type being established in other areas of the country where they are not now available. I think we have demonstrated that a program can be developed that provides a high-quality of medical care and that does not have great cost duplications. I think it gives great opportunity, as we look at some of the problems facing American medicine and the American economy."

Kaiser has started spreading eastward from the West Coast

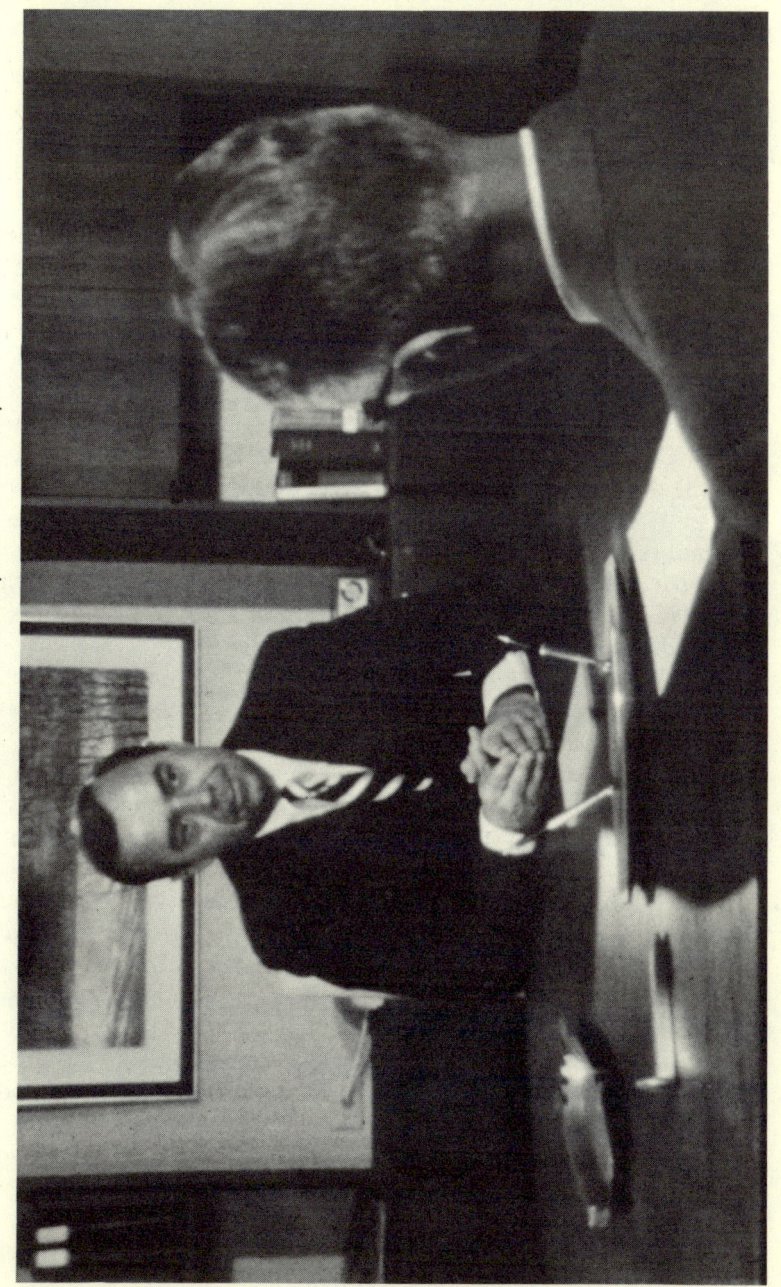

"No loss in the doctor-patient relationship...."

to Denver and to Cleveland but, fearing to become too big, does not plan to spread much further. But other group plans have sprung up, such as New York City's Health Insurance Plan (HIP), with three-quarters of a million members. Its growth has been impeded by not owning its own facilities, but it has recently acquired LaGuardia Hospital in Queens. With the active encouragement of Blue Cross-Blue Shield and of the commercial insurance companies which have committed themselves to pushing for "soundly conceived changes," some medical schools are being encouraged to create new group programs. Today, more than 6 million Americans are enrolled in such plans.

One of the newest programs is the Harvard Community Health Plan for the Boston area, supported by Blue Cross and ten insurance companies, including giants like Metropolitan, Prudential, and Equitable, which actually canvass subscriptions among their clients signed up for other health plans. They are hoping to develop a model that Blue Cross and the insurance companies can use as a prototype.

Dr. Jerome Pollack of Harvard, who designed the model, told us that "group practice is an idea whose time is not only ripe, but overripe." He said:

"We need physicians working in groups who can see up to one-fifth more patients than they could treat individually. We have a great shortage of doctors, and group practice has at last become respectable when it is no longer enough. We need not only groups of doctors, but medical teams with other skills. We need skills not yet even identified, people who will be trained, find a place in the health-care system and relieve the doctor by doing some things better than the doctor now does.

"We need to tie this immediately to the financing because it isn't enough to have a group if that group isn't associated with a population that has agreed to get its medical care from the group, and if the group isn't committed to taking care of all the needs of that population. That is why group practice must be tied in with prepayment.

"I visualize an expansion not only of Kaiser's plans, but

much more advanced plans starting from that premise, plans picked up by such university medical schools as Harvard, Johns Hopkins, and Yale, spread by insurance company and Blue Cross prepayment plans. I foresee plans covering millions of people."

The medical establishment, though far from enthusiastic, is veering from outright opposition to reluctant tolerance of the prepaid-practice concept. Dr. Gerald Dorman, president of the AMA, stated it cautiously:

"Fee for service is not necessarily the only way to do practice. That depends on the physician and on the situation in which he is. There is nothing unethical as to whether it is fee-for-service or is paid for in some other way. . . . Don't let me give the impression that the solo, fee-for-service is the only ethical way to practice medicine. On the whole, though, I think it is the best way. . . .

"I think that in the large centers solo practice very often will fade out—not by fiat, but that's the way it's going to work. . . . We will develop towards a different system, yes! This I believe. But I don't think we need—and I think it would be a catastrophe—to have what's going on now wiped out and an entirely new system put in suddenly. . . .

"I don't think it will be all on a capitation basis, a salary basis. Some doctors like that way of doing business. . . . There are other doctors who feel that they produce better if they realize that it is on a fee-for-service basis. And they say all doctors are prima donnas! Whether you like it or not, we wouldn't have gone into medicine had we not been prima donnas."

Dr. Fein says that the behavior of prima donnas can be changed—by economic pressure.

"We have learned from prepaid group health programs," he says, "that hospital days can be cut sixty percent with no reduction in quality—and probably some improvement. But, as long as we have the single practitioner making a set of little decisions, we will continue to have problems. In this field, in contrast with other fields, the consumer has not been the critical decision maker. It is the physician, and he is ultimately the point of leverage. It is his behavior we will have to change.

"There are two ways of forcing people to recognize necessity—coercion and incentive. I would like to see us use incentive to get more responsible behavior from the private sector.

"We are entitled to get our money's worth when the Government spends our tax dollars. This means that the Government is going to have to take sides. If group practice is an efficient way of delivering medical care, then the Government will have to stimulate group practice.

"When the Government goes to buy an airplane it says, 'This is what we want. Who is ready to deliver it and at what price?' One could imagine the Government saying, in the health field, 'We have a population we would like to cover. These are the services the population needs. Is there anybody who wants to offer these services, and at what price? Is Kaiser ready to bid? Is the Harvard Community Health Plan ready to bid? Is Prudential, Equitable, who are now getting into the field?'

"I think that only on a prepaid group basis is one really going to come to grips with the problem. But this will require a Government policy that is not neutral between efficiency and inefficiency."

As Dr. Fein spoke, within the Government wheels were already turning in this direction. The Federal Task Force on Medicaid and Related Problems, working for almost a year to chart a route out of the morass, reported, "We strongly support the principle of providing an option for Medicare and Medicaid beneficiaries that would permit them to elect to receive health services through a single organization in a coordinated manner, financed through prepaid capitation. The Health Maintenance Organization proposal constitutes an important step towards possible long-range improvements in the organization and delivery of health services."

Few realized that almost three-and-a-half years before this recommendation to the Nixon Administration, another report to President Johnson on medical care prices had urged virtually the same thing—amend the law to allow Medicaid beneficiaries to use prepaid group practice plans... encourage the states to foster such plans . . . provide "seed money" to encourage the development of medical teams.

The Johnson Administration had passed over the recommendation in silence. Three years and billions of dollars later, the climate had changed. Robert Finch, then HEW secretary, said, "We must promote diversity, choice, and healthy competition in American medicine if we are to escape from the grip of spiraling costs." Dr. James Cavanaugh, Deputy Assistant Secretary for Health, called it "the most important proposal to come along since Medicare and Medicaid were enacted in 1965."

Reacting to the pressures, the AMA made some grudging concessions. The 1970 meeting of its House of Delegates in Chicago recognized "the need for multiple methods of delivering medical services," and said that the AMA "advocates factual investigation and objective experimentation in new methods of delivery of health care, while still maintaining faith and trust in the private practice of medicine and pride in its accomplishments." It could, however, still not quite bring itself to endorse directly "prepaid group practice." But the Federal Government was no longer waiting for the AMA.

HEW issued new regulations giving Medicaid beneficiaries "freedom of choice" among providers of health services, including "organizations offering medical services on a prepaid or membership basis." Legislation was introduced to give Medicare beneficiaries the same option and to permit contracts to be signed for comprehensive services and preventive care.

But if there is any large-scale response among the more than 30 million beneficiaries of Medicare and Medicaid, the existing prepaid plans will not have the capacity to absorb them. Unlike the insurance companies, the Nixon Administration showed no immediate signs that it was willing to spend large amounts to help foster the HMOs it praised so highly. The first Government money to come for creation of new organizations was a half-million dollars from the Office of Economic Opportunity to organizations in Memphis and

Milwaukee to create "innovative prepaid group practices to provide comprehensive health care for the poor." The guidelines required physicians wishing to join to bring their paying patients with them.

The concept of an annual fee to an organized group for comprehensive "Keep Well" services has begun to take hold in a Government growing desperate about the cost of inefficiency. Crisis has begun to force change. And other innovations were claiming attention.

CHAPTER VIII
BRINGING THE
POOR INTO THE HEALTH SYSTEM

"When the 30 million poor perceive," said Dr. John Knowles of Massachusetts General Hospital, "that we are not meeting their right of health, I fear a confrontation with the medical establishment, the kind of destructive confrontation that occurred in New York City when people perceived that their educational system was not fulfilling their rights."

Nowhere does the Constitution guarantee a right to health—as it *does* provide for an educational system. Yet the right to health has become a rallying cry, a theme that kept cropping up in our interviews. It is vigorously asserted by the activists and bridled at by the health establishment as a menacing, radical slogan like "Power to the People."

It came up when Rashi Fein said, "We say people have a right to education, and then somebody goes out and makes sure that there is a school and there are teachers. But if the people of western Massachusetts have a right to medical care and there are no doctors, no one says that it is our responsibility to see that there are physicians there."

It came up when Professor Harry Becker said, "This question of health care as a right.... We have all kinds of mixed feelings about it. We'll say pick up a man off the street with a bleeding wound, or a child in a lead-poisoning coma, but we find it difficult to face up to the proper diagnosis and follow-through for children who may have indications of lead-poisoning. We say, on the one hand, that health care is a right, but on the other hand, we create all kinds of barriers in getting there."

It came up when Dr. Knowles said, "Medicine in this country has evolved in the last half-century as a highly technical, highly scientific, extremely interesting pursuit for doctors and institutions.... But in their rush to acquire more knowledge and to carry out this high-cost curative care, they have neglected the extension of their services to communities within their reach to prevent disease or detect it in its incipiency."

The "right to health" is raised constantly in the context of a general indictment of American medicine as self-centered rather than people-centered. But it is raised with particular force when the health of the poor is discussed. For the hard core of America's health problem is close to the hard core of America's poverty problem. Even if the medical industry reorganized itself enough to curtail its prices and the waiting-time in the doctor's office, that would not necessarily solve the problem of the millions without access to the doctor's office, many without even a notion of what it would be like to be healthy.

In Boston, for example, 350 of 1,000 persons between sixteen and twenty-one, examined in the ghetto, were found to have undiagnosed diseases. Dr. Knowles gave some of the reasons, "Geographic limitations... transportation... simple inaccessibility to health workers . . . lack of knowledge of how to get into the system."

"Many families, living in the midst of poverty and disease," he said, "don't expect anything else. In certain sections of the city, people simply don't have money or available transportation to get across the city to a health facility. Many think that if they come to this hospital and can't pay, they won't be cared for, and so they don't bother coming. Some go to municipal hospitals and sit all day and then go home, afraid of losing jobs because the boss will think they are deadbeats. A mother waits for her husband to come home to take care of the other children while she takes one to the clinic, and then finds there is no evening clinic. . . ."

Boston is no exception. Nationally, a child born to poor parents has twice the average risk of dying before he becomes thirty-five as a child born of middle-class parents. There is twice as much illness among the poor, four times as much chronic illness, three times as much heart disease, seven times as many eye defects, five times as much mental retardation and nervous disorders.

So, it dawned on us that more than theory is involved in the debate over the "right to health." It has become a kind of demarcation line in the struggle over reform of the nation's health system. Because it implies a commitment to serve all Americans, it implies a commitment to change the health system so that it *can* serve all Americans. Some of those in positions of responsibility are reluctant to concede the right, if for no other reason than that they do not know how it is to be fulfilled.

An independent critic like Dr. Becker can say, "Health care has to be in the same category as education. It's got to be available to everybody on the same basis. We give lip service to health care as a right, but in reality, when it comes to delivering that service, we find various ways of setting up constraints and barriers."

Walter McNerney's task force on health problems of the poor can say, "The first big idea is that all consumers should have access to health care without hardship and, as far as possible, with some voice in how it is planned and some choice of how it is furnished."

And, further, it can say, "The task force, along with what is possibly a majority in the health professions, and certainly a majority of the country, considers the recent Federal enactments as intending that access to basic medical care shall be a right or entitlement of all citizens. It is the position of the task force that the right or entitlement is not fulfilled when millions in the population do not know about or cannot get to the places where some care is available to deprived populations, or when millions who do get to such places are given a kind of service that is woefully inferior by every standard known to man and doctor. Neither is the right or entitlement honored just because physicians and hospital administrators can say, 'We never turn away patients.' However virtuous the declaration may make the doctors and hospital people feel, it does nothing to make good the right or entitlement for those who never get within sight of a doctor's office."

But those who are asked to deliver the goods speak in more guarded terms.

Mark Berke, president of the American Hospital Association, told us, "If we really talk about health as a right of the American people, we're talking about something with fantastic overtones and undertones in terms of organization of health services. As people perceive this as a right, we're

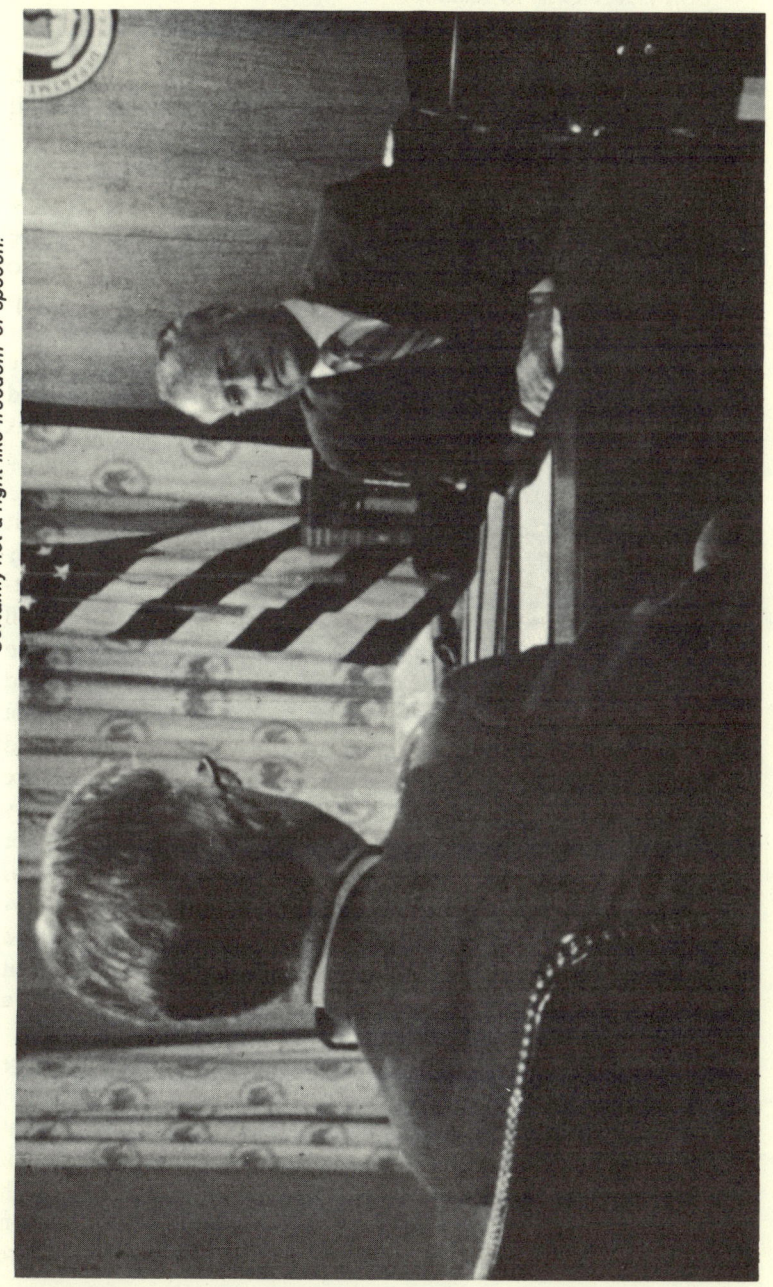

"Certainly not a right like freedom of speech."

finding that more and more are coming who had really neglected their health. . . . We're dealing with an ever-increasing number of serious cases and complicated cases, requiring longer hospital stays until we can get them under control."

The Nixon Administration has made no commitment on the right to health. And when I pressed John Veneman, undersecretary of HEW, on the subject in an interview, he said that he saw health care as a responsibility for Government on all levels—local, state, and Federal—but "certainly not a right like freedom of speech."

The American Medical Association, until recently, took the position that health care is "not a right, but a privilege." Now, somewhat more defensive, the current American Medical Association president, Dr. Gerald Dorman, fenced on the issue in an interview which went like this:

"I don't hold any position as to right or privilege. I think it's the obligation of the physician to take care of his patient."

"And whose obligation to pay for it?"

"This is primarily the obligation of the patient, secondarily of his family, thirdly of the local area, town, or city, and the Federal Government, finally."

Dr. Dorman said, "We want to see the poor treated the same as everybody else in the country—as private patients so that they can get the best possible care."

This, in fact, is the premise on which Medicaid was based—the Federal and state Governments providing the money so that the poor could get to the doctor's office, without tampering with the system. That, it is now generally agreed, has not worked. At stupendous cost, it has reached only a third of the poor with inadequate care.

What has become clear is that no carpet of money—even if there were enough to subsidize an inefficient system—will transport the poor to the doctor's office. A whole new approach is needed, an approach going beyond what is needed to improve health services for the more affluent.

In our investigation we saw one such approach being tried, with some early but dramatic signs of success.

On Chicago's West Side, one section listed among twenty-

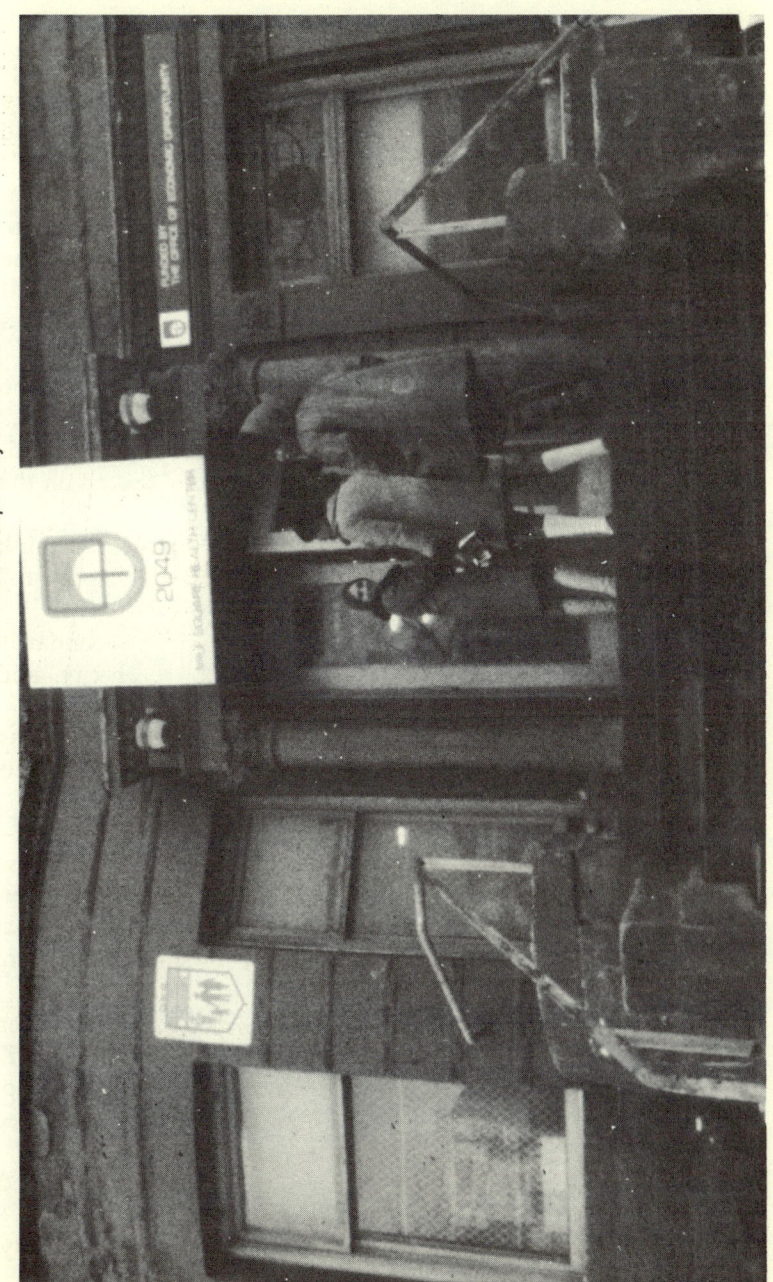

"... well accepted by the residents."

four areas of concentrated poverty is called Mile Square. It is an area that *is* roughly a mile square, with about 25,000 inhabitants, ninety percent of them Black, thirteen percent of the workers unemployed, twenty-five percent of the residents getting public assistance, forty percent of them living in public housing.

In this section of decaying tenements and malnourished children, infant mortality is 60 percent higher than Chicago's average, tuberculosis 200 percent higher, and venereal disease 550 percent higher. And many of the people had not seen a doctor in years.

In 1967, at the request of the community, something new came to Mile Square. It was one of those new-fangled neighborhood health centers with which the anti-poverty agency, Office of Economic Opportunity, had started experimenting. St. Luke's Presbyterian Hospital contracted to set up the medical organization, but it was more than a clinic. What made it novel was not that it provided free care, but that, under one roof in their own neighborhood, it provided most of what the residents needed, both treatment and preventive examinations. It took care of the whole family, and kept records of the whole family to insure continuity. It didn't wait for people to come, but sent staff members recruited from the community to seek out residents who might need help. And people from the neighborhood not only filled jobs in the center, but served on its board to set policy. It was meant to be not only a facility to provide for their health, but also *their* health facility.

Much more could be said about this as an instrument for social change, but we are talking about health. By its third year Mile Square Health Center was seeing 18,000 of the 25,000 residents, giving them everything from prenatal care to mental health treatment. Those who had to go to the hospital went to St. Luke's Presbyterian with special plastic cards to make sure they would get proper attention. And the locally recruited, locally trained community health aides, a new breed of cat, made 23,000 home visits in a year.

Cold-eyed investigators from the General Accounting Office, the financial watchdog of Congress, came to see if this was a boon or a boondoggle. They picked forty-eight records from the file at random and asked the patients what the Health Center had done for them. The GAO reported the responses: Thirty-eight said their health had been improved; ten said conditions were found that they had not known about; thirty said they received better care than elsewhere; forty-six said they visited the center at least four times; forty-four said they would come again; forty said they were very satisfied with the care received; and forty-three said they received attention with reasonable speed.

The GAO team concluded: "The center made medical services readily available to its target-area residents, many of whom received little or only fragmented care prior to the existence of the center, and the center was well-accepted by the residents."

The GAO noted bureaucratic problems—such as whether all who received free care were poor enough to qualify for it. (Dr. Rashi Fein scoffed at the problem, saying, "If one builds a water fountain in the middle of the desert, one does not have to ask whether each person coming to the fountain really needs a drink; one can assume that.") But the GAO also noted a measure of success in an area where few successes have been achieved before.

There are difficulties that Dr. Joyce Lashoff, the co-director, talked to Correspondent George Herman about. "We are seeing almost 300 patients a day in a building that we didn't think could accommodate more than 100. There are times when we have five doctors and four examining rooms for them to work in. We've extended hours into the evening and Saturday."

But these are mainly problems of growth. Dr. Lashoff said, "In three years you don't solve all the problems. But we are caring for people, and they are getting a much higher volume of care than they ever had before. Infant mortality for the patients to whom we have given prenatal care has dropped remarkably. We have seen families and patients who have been neglected over periods of time that we've been able to get functioning again. We have seen mentally retarded children who received no care at all before this center was opened—children discovered by our aides and nurses.

"There are problems that it's going to take a lot of long, hard work to be able to solve in a community like this. But certainly the center is looked to by the community as its source of medical care now. And we are seeing changes in their patterns of care in this population.

"We think that we will be able to show that we can decrease hospitalization rates, improve the health of the community, hopefully decrease infant mortality rates. We can't show all of that right off in a couple of years. But, as an experiment, this has proven that the community accepts, wants, will utilize medical care, and that we can recruit the staff to deliver the medical care. I would say that it works!"

The name of the OEO program that pays for the Mile Square Health Center is, by no accident, "Healthright." It is a holdover from the Johnsonian "Great Society," but, because of its reputation as the most successful of the anti-poverty programs and its wide support in Congress, has been taken to the Nixon Administration's bosom.

No trumpets sounded when "Healthright" was born, almost as an afterthought, in the early days of the Johnson "war on poverty." In the planning of that war, health was not originally envisaged as one of the battlegrounds.

But it began to dawn on the anti-poverty warriors that job training made little sense for a man physically unable to work, and that innovations in education would do little for sick children. As community action groups around the country spelled out their needs, some of them included requests for help in medical projects. The OEO began to wonder whether it shouldn't be doing something more comprehensive and original about health care.

By coincidence, two doctors in Boston were devising an experimental plan for a new kind of health center for the poor. Dr. H. Jack Geiger, a specialist in social medicine in under-developed countries, had worked with an urban and a rural health center for poor Blacks in South Africa, on lines

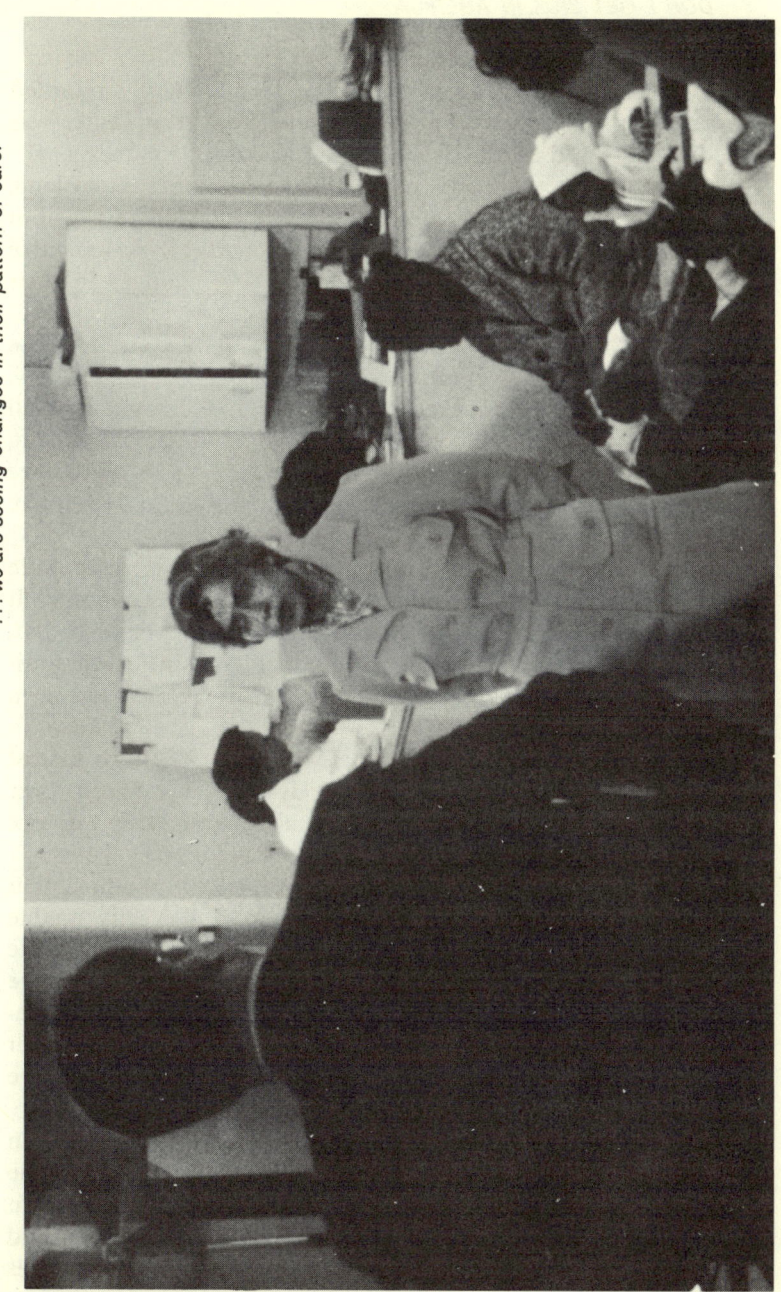

"... we are seeing changes in their pattern of care."

charted by Dr. John Grant of the Rockefeller Foundation. Dr. Geiger's idea was that what had worked for the poor in developing countries of Africa and Latin America was adaptable to the poor of the United States. He was joined by Dr. Count Gibson, Jr., a Georgia-born internist.

They brought their plan to the U.S. Public Health Service in Washington, which bewilderedly referred them to the new anti-poverty agency. The OEO was interested, but dismissed their modest request for a $30,000 planning grant as small potatoes for an agency under pressure to get its first hundred million to work.

Encouraged to think big—in terms of hundreds of thousands and a center not a study—they thought even bigger and returned with a proposal for a $1.25 million grant for two health centers, one in the urban North, the other in the rural South. It was accepted.

On a spit of land in Boston Harbor, built over a one-time city dump, stood Columbia Point, a public housing area with some 6,000 residents, roughly half Whites and half non-Whites. More than two hours away from the nearest hospital by inadequate transportation, it was an ideal place for a new health facility.

Here, at the end of 1965, sponsored by the Tufts University School of Medicine, rose the Columbia Point Health Center—first in the nation to offer the poor comprehensive, one-stop service, with a full range of preventive and home care, with new kinds of neighborhood-trained semi-professionals like "home health aides," "family health workers" and "clinic aides," working with teams of family physicians and specialists.

Health services had not only come to the neighborhood, but had also become a part of the neighborhood, no longer alien and remote. A former welfare recipient, now a family health worker, could persuade a woman to come to the health center and bring her children. In the first year, more than ninety percent of the children in the area visited the center. Within two years, the need of Columbia Point residents for hospital care had dropped an astonishing eighty percent. In its third year, the center was being used by seventy-eight percent of the people in the neighborhood.

It was not surprising that the center would attract those without health care and those who had been relying on hospital out-patient clinics. But it also attracted those who had been seeing private doctors. An evaluation report said, "While the private practitioner is widely seen as synonymous with high quality of care and the personal manner in which it is rendered, it appears that only a small minority of *poor* patients have had such a positive experience with private medical practice."

In the rural South it was harder. In Bolivar County, in the Mississippi Delta country, where windows of shacks are stuffed with paper and unemployment runs as high as seventy-five percent, it was hard even to get Blacks to believe that help from outside was conceivable. In Mound Bayou, oldest all-Black community in the nation, the Tufts-Delta Health Center was started in a remodeled church parsonage, with examining rooms in former bedrooms and a laboratory in the former kitchen.

"We found people with seemingly endless unmet medical needs," Dr. Geiger recalls. "Some stark conditions had existed, untreated or undiagnosed, for decades. Some were straight out of the 19th Century textbooks of infectious disease."

Since then the health center has moved twice and now is in its permanent home, two large buildings with a staff of 180. Ninety percent of the non-medical staff are Black Mississippians, and the ratio of Black professionals is increasing, thanks partly to the efforts of the health center in sending local residents to universities to learn medicine, nursing, and allied professions.

By the middle of 1970, the health center had more than 12,000 patients—almost ninety percent of the area's population—and was seeing 4,700 patients a month in the center, which does not include the hundreds aided in field visits. The northern Bolivar County poor also had what their city cousins might envy—two doctors on call every night. There was extra food for infants, pregnant women, and nursing mothers. The infant mortality rate had dropped from seventy to thirty per thousand—"a pretty respectable figure," says Dr. Geiger.

From the center radiated a network of village health associations. For the 14,000 poor Blacks of this Delta area, a health center had not only changed their physical well-being, but revolutionized their way of life. It helped communities organize water supply to replace drinking from drainage ditches. It built new privies from the wood of abandoned shacks. It set up a unit to clean up garbage dumps and kill rats. It went so far as to help organize a cooperative farm that now employs 800 families and produces a million pounds of food a year for its members.

There are forty-nine neighborhood health centers around the country now, including one for Mexican-Americans in Alviso, California, and one for Chippewa Indians on the Red Lake Reservation of Minnesota. They operate from storefronts in The Bronx and from wooden frames in Kentucky. The biggest of them is in Watts, Los Angeles, built over the rubble of the 1965 riots. And in Watts, when summer brings talk of more riots, one can hear a militant say, "We'll burn everything down—everything except the health center. That's ours!"

The OEO has put $300 million into the experimental health centers, that money supplemented by other Government programs and by Medicare and Medicaid reimbursement. Now that they are no longer considered as experimental, HEW is starting to take over the centers at which its Public Health Service blinked when they were first proposed.

Dr. Geiger says the nation needs 800 such centers. The Federal Task Force on Health recommended, "Priority should be given to development of organized primary health-care services in neighborhoods."

Short of 800 comprehensive centers that would heal, employ, and involve the people of the neighborhood, the experiment has had an impact in promoting the general idea of bringing a package of health services to the poor.

In some cases, as with Massachusetts General Hospital,

it takes the simple form of putting branch clinics out into the ghetto. In some areas it takes the form of an adaptation of group practice. In the Shaw District of Washington, D.C., private physicians and the local health department have created a "group practice without walls"—a community health center, plus additional services provided in doctors' offices.

Under the life insurance industry's $2 billion program for the inner city and the Federal Government's Model Cities program, loans and grants are being used to build ghetto health centers.

Health centers for the poor, like prepaid group practice, are potential building blocks of a modernized health system that can make the "right to health" a reality. There remains the question of what kind of roof will cover these blocks—what will be the national plan for health.

CHAPTER IX
HOW THEY DO IT OVER THERE

DON'T GET SICK IN AMERICA

An American's pride was wounded when Johan van der Sande, after returning to Holland for health benefits he could not afford in California, said, "America is a good place to live if you're healthy, but don't get sick in America!"

More important is the question of how smaller and poorer countries manage to provide the kind of health security that in this country would empty Fort Knox, fill the hospitals, and prostrate our doctors with exhaustion—or so we are told. What is this "national health insurance" that gave Mr. Van der Sande his artificial kidney and all the rest of his treatment for a premium of $24 a month?

It is no mystery. Holland's health-security programs is one of the widely-varying systems that have grown up in welfare-conscious Europe, long sensitive to the economic risks of illness. Holland, where "medical clubs" date back to the Middle Ages, probably has the longest history of voluntary health insurance in the world. In 1941, the hundred insurance plans were coordinated under a national health insurance law, which has been updated several times, most recently in 1968.

It was in 1968 that Mr. Van der Sande, along with everyone else living in the Netherlands, became eligible for reimbursement for "special" or "prolonged" illness. A person need not apply for this insurance until he needs it. The plan is financed by a 0.4 percent payroll tax, with employers contributing. This insurance plan was the latest addition to the national health protection program, which was codified in the Health Insurance Act of 1966. The act provided compulsory coverage for wage-earners, the aging, and the disabled, paid largely by employers through a 7.2 percent payroll tax. It is not a universal system. About half the population is insured compulsorily, and another twenty percent voluntarily. The remaining thirty percent—including principally the rural population, the very poor, and the very rich—must depend on their own resources, on voluntary insurance, or on charity.

For the seventy percent of the Dutch population who are covered, it works this way: Under general regulations set by the Government, the local insurance plans contract with hospitals and professionals. Doctors are paid on a capitation

HOW THEY DO IT OVER THERE

basis—each doctor receives a fixed annual amount for every person registered with him for care. The beneficiary chooses his own family doctor, but he can only see a specialist to whom he is referred by his doctor. His insurance covers hospital treatment up to one year per illness, plus drugs and a variety of other benefits, and dental care under some conditions.

The Dutch system could no more be copied by the United States than the Swedish, the German, or the British. European health insurance systems are rooted in European history, and each in its own history. In the countries influenced by the French Revolution and the Napoleonic conquests, there was an early tendency toward state intervention. In the Germany of the 1880s, social insurance developed as part of Chancellor Bismarck's struggle to undercut the rising Socialist movement. European countries have, on the whole, long been comfortable with a welfare-state approach, still a subject of controversy in the United States. Whatever the historic reasons, European countries *have* organized general access to health care through comprehensive national plans, and they have lessons to teach the United States, which is still seeking the means of accomplishing that aim.

The lessons percolate with difficulty through a fog of emotion that clouds the issue. Many American tourists who have fallen ill in Europe have returned with stories about cheap or free care. Many American doctors who have made postman's holiday inspections of health care in Europe have returned with horror stories of medicine in bureaucratic chains. It may be time to set down a few of the basic facts about the organization of health care on a national basis in Europe.

There are three ways of paying doctors under European plans sometimes used in combination with each other.

Fee-for-Service—a fee for each procedure, sometimes paid by the patient subject to reimbursement, sometimes paid by the Government or an intermediary.

Capitation—a fixed annual payment for every person on

a doctor's list of patients, regardless of how often the patient sees his doctor in a year. A variation is "case payment," a fixed sum paid only for persons who become ill.

Salary—a fixed payment to the doctor, based not on how many patients he sees, but on his professional rank and the amount of time he gives.

With this brief glossary as a guide, here, briefly summarized, is how other countries provide health care.

Great Britain

National Health Insurance is administered by the Department of Health and Social Security. Eighty-five percent of the cost is borne by the Government, with a small contribution by workers and employers. It covers all residents, plus most visitors. Physicians operating on a panel system, receive a fixed schedule of fees from National Health Service for special services. General practitioners are reimbursed on a capitation basis. The National Health Service runs a system of national hospitals, directly administered by the Department of Health, with their personnel, including doctors, on salary. Health centers, clinics, and extended-care facilities are operated by county councils.

Sweden

The sickness insurance scheme is supervised by the National Social Insurance Board under the general supervision of the Ministry of Social Affairs. Insurance is compulsory (children under sixteen are covered by their parents' insurance). Foreign workers and other foreign residents who are registered for census purposes are entitled to the same benefits as citizens. The National Board of Health and Welfare supervises the medical personnel, the hospitals, and the pharmacies, and it has direct control over the state mental hospitals, the state pharmaceutical laboratory, and the state institutions for forensic medicine.

Most hospitals are owned and operated by public authorities, primarily at the county level. The regional social insurance offices pay seventy-five percent of the physician's services up to certain limits listed in published fee schedules approved by the Government after negotiation with the Swedish Medical Association. Individuals have a free choice among doctors, and all doctors participate in the program.

West Germany

Health insurance is under the general supervision of the Ministry of Labor and Social Affairs and is administered through state insurance offices. There are about 2,000 local, occupational, and other funds, managed by elected representatives of insured persons and employers and organized into state and national federations. It is compulsory for all wage and salary workers below a certain earnings level to be enrolled in a health fund, not necessarily a public one.

Doctors are associated with individual funds and are paid by them on a fee-for-service basis. The most common criterion for payment is a nationwide fee schedule, arrived at by the social security carriers and the organization of sickness insurance doctors, and subject to approval of the Ministry. Hospitals are maintained by public authorities (state and local governments, universities, and insurance institutions), and by private organizations (churches, trade unions, and private owners [in the case of sanitariums]), with national subsidies available.

France

The national health insurance fund operates under the general supervision of the Ministry of Social Affairs. Management control is exercised through sixteen regional Social Security Fund offices which have authority to negotiate hospital and medical fee schedules with regional professional associations. All wage and salary earners, farmers, craftsmen, self-employed and retired persons, are covered. Aliens working in France are entitled to the same benefits as citizens.

All doctors participate in the program. The rates of payment are fixed on a fee-for-service basis by agreement between the Social Security Administration and the medical associations. All public hospitals and a number of private institutions approved by the Social Security Administration participate. Health insurance covers seventy-five percent of outpatient medical and dental bills, eighty percent of medical fees, laboratory tests and hospitalization, and seventy-five percent of most pharmaceutical prescriptions.

Canada

Canada is included only briefly because it just recently joined the national health insurance ranks. Health insurance operates under a joint federal-provincial system. The Department of National Health and Welfare shares costs and provides consultative services. The Federal Government provides about half of the medical insurance costs of the participating provinces. The basic aim of the provincial systems is universal coverage of all residents, with a waiting period for nonresidents.

Most public general hospitals have been approved for inclusion in the hospital insurance system. Selected private hospitals providing special and convalescent care have been approved for payment on a contract basis in most provinces. The method of paying physicians varies from province to province.

The Communist Way

The system of health care in the Communist bloc, with its centralization, rigidity, and lack of opportunity for free choice for either doctor or patient, is not a system the United States is likely to emulate. This is not to deny its phenomenal success in providing easy access to health care for a vast population in widely dispersed areas.

In the Communist-ruled countries, a Ministry of Health operates a network of hospitals and dispensaries. Physicians and other professionals are on salary, although they can supplement their incomes by private "moonlighting." Health care is financed from the state budget, and patients pay only a share of drug costs. Patients are assigned to the nearest facilities, like it or not. If not, they can, at their own expense, have recourse to the moonlighters. That is the only time they are likely to see a doctor in a private office.

For the salaried doctors, incentive payments are closely geared to the goals of the regime. For example, a bonus may be paid to a physician in an industrial location if absenteeism at the factory is low. This encourages prevention of illness; it also sometimes encourages "doctored" reports to underestimate the extent of illness. The doctors, a large majority of them women, are relatively poorly paid—often earning little more than skilled workers. Individual practice has virtually disappeared. It is not an ideal situation for doctors; it does, however, despite long waits, excessive paper work, and other inconveniences, serve the community. Some eighty percent of the 230 million Soviet citizens visit their polyclinics every year for free care and check-ups.

It is not likely that any other system would have worked as well in a country which started with a shortage of medical resources. This is why the Soviet national health service concept is being emulated in many under-developed countries, but it would be considered repugnant by Americans, doctors and patients alike.

The British Way

The National Health Service, in effect since 1948, entitles everyone in the British Isles to basically free health care, financed principally by the Government.

A general practitioner receives a capitation payment of about $2.50 a year for every patient registered with him, regardless of how much treatment he gives that patient. His "panel" is limited to 3,500 patients, considered the maximum he can feasibly handle. The average family doctor has 2,470 patients on his list, and sees about 200 a week. Ninety-seven percent of British residents are registered with National Health Service doctors, though they are free to see doctors privately outside the national system. They are also free to choose their doctors, although, in practice, they tend to stick with the doctors most conveniently available to home or place of work.

The physician, except for working in a situation of virtual government monopoly of his services, is independent. He usually operates from his own office and with his own staff.

He is encouraged, by extra pay incentives, to work with groups of physicians, but he is not compelled to do so. The British doctor is a busy man, seeing almost twice as many patients a week as his American colleague. Yet house calls, on their way to extinction in the United States, are still a large part of the British doctor's work.

The British doctor is rewarded for doing things which are considered socially useful. He gets extra pay for treating a person over sixty-five, for making night calls, for treating transients, for providing maternity care, for giving preventive care, and for moving to a remote area short of physicians.

For all the grousing about over-long waits and over-speedy service, there is no doubt that the British use their health service. Three out of four consult their family doctors at least once a year—on the average, three to four times per person.

Because of British tradition rather than because of the National Health Service, once the patient goes to the hospital he is out of the hands of his family doctor. In the nationalized hospital, the system is different. The independent physician paid by capitation is replaced by a fully salaried staff in publicly operated institutions, all integrated within a single system and with easy transfer from one to the other for specialized services.

In Britain, getting into the hospital is sometimes difficult since admission is based on a waiting list. It may take a week or two in fairly urgent cases, up to a year for elective surgery. At any given time a nationwide waiting list of half a million is not uncommon.

There is less hospitalization (ten percent of the population) than in the United States (fifteen percent) not only because it is hard to get in, but also because the outpatient departments, integrated in the hospitals, screen applicants and provide considerable testing and treatment that often make admission unnecessary. Although the American's average hospital stay is shorter than his British cousin's, this does not necessarily mean greater efficiency. Britons could not get into the hospital for "tests" or "observation," as Americans frequently do because our hospital-oriented, private insurance makes it cheaper to do so. The British National Health Service has its flaws. The general practitioner, who is the backbone of the system, regards himself as underpaid, and the family doctors are in a constant state of latent rebellion that leads to large-scale emigration.

Doctors also complain of the deadening effects of having to refer cases to specialists and to hospitals. There are complaints about paperwork, and about under-financing of the system. But few of the doctors who agitate for improvements in the system and even fewer patients would today want to replace that system.

One British doctor told American interviewer Donald Drake of the Philadelphia *Inquirer*, "I can certainly understand why your doctors don't want socialized medicine. But it is beyond me how they have convinced their patients and their government that it would not be in the public's interest." A British medical writer said, "In the American system the primary concern is for the doctor and not the patient. In Britain, the concern is for the patient."

A natural question is how Britain, with its National Health Service, stacks up against free-wheeling America in costs and quality of health care. Britain, in fact, spends relatively less for health than the United States does—in 1961, 4 percent of its Gross National Product against 5.5 percent in the United States. In 1965, Britain spent only 71 percent as much as the U.S., in Gross National Product terms. As to quality, this was the analysis of HEW:

"The smaller share of Gross National Product going to medical care in the United Kingdom does not necessarily indicate a level of medical services inferior to that of the United States. Since, in relation to per capita national income, net incomes of doctors, hospital costs, and drug costs all seem to be lower in the United Kingdom than in the United States, a smaller portion of Gross National Product would suffice to provide the same degree of health care prevailing in the United States. . . . In terms of crude criteria often used for this purpose (infant mortality rates, standardized death rates, physician-population ratio, and hospital bed-population ratio) the effectiveness of the two programs seems to be roughly the same."

The Swedish Way

Sweden, as in so many other fields, chose the middle way in national health insurance, but this was after a bruising struggle with organized medicine reminiscent of the controversy confronting the United States. There were other parallels. As in this country, voluntary insurance was widespread, covering two-thirds of the population, and Government programs cared for the aged and the poor, though inadequately.

In 1947 a government commission proposed a national health service based entirely on full-time salaried doctors. The enraged Swedish Medical Association advocated preservation of the fee-for-service principle and enlisted the support of business groups and conservative political parties in fighting the national health plan. The outcome, a law passed in 1953 which went into effect in 1955, was a compromise—a national health insurance system that made medical service available to most of the population with minimal changes in the working conditions of doctors.

There were more years of storm and stress with the medical association, but finally the dust settled and the system that emerged was this:

Everyone sixteen and older, with an income exceeding a certain minimum, pays an annual insurance premium, based on his income and the area where he lives (to take into account variations in costs among regions). For this premium he and his dependents receive benefits amounting to seventy-five percent of the official fee for each medical procedure. The fee schedule is relatively short and simple as such schedules go. The patient pays the doctor, gets a receipt, and the regional insurance office reimburses him for seventy-five percent of it. This, it should be noted, is one of the least generous formulas in Europe, but it reflects the drastic shortage of physicians in Sweden and the desire to discourage overutilization. There has been such a scarcity of doctors in Sweden—thanks to the medical association's success in holding down the number of medical students—that physicians are booked far in advance. Many in need of care shop through the "yellow pages" of their telephone directories for names of new physicians.

In practice, thanks to the competition for care, average reimbursement is substantially less than seventy-five percent. The doctors who practice privately (1,200 of the total of 9,200) set their own fees, but reimbursement is still on the basis of the official fee. Thus, many patients get as little as fifty percent of their doctors' bills refunded.

Because of the difficulty in getting treatment, many Swedes have been sent to the out-patient clinics of hospitals. There, until recently, hospital doctors, though working on salaries, could treat out-patients on a fee-for-service basis. Doctors were thus making a profit on the use of hospital clinics as their offices. Under a reform introduced in 1970, a flat fee of $1.33 was fixed for any outpatient treatment in the hospital. The hospital doctors were to receive none of this fee, but were given a twenty percent increase in salary as a consolation. The effect of this cut-rate care has been to make hospitals more popular for ambulatory treatment than in most countries.

Hospitalization, under the Swedish insurance system, is free in public wards, as are all needed surgery, medical treatment, laboratory and X-ray tests, and drugs. There are additional personally paid charges for patients who want semi-private or private rooms. There are also some surviving private hospitals, where the patient pays all costs, but so few are willing to do so that private hospitals now represent fewer than three percent of beds in Swedish general hospitals.

As in Britain, when a patient goes to the hospital, he loses contact with his family doctor and comes under the care of a salaried hospital physician. This is more a product of tradition than of the insurance system. In fact, Swedish medical authorities, concerned about the results of this separation, have started rotating general practitioners through the hospitals to catch up with new techniques.

As in Britain, there is usually a long wait for outpatient

care, and a longer wait for admission to a hospital bed. There is an average wait of three months for non-emergency operations, and the hospital waiting list, at any given time, is about 80,000—a two-month case load.

The main burden of financing the Swedish health insurance system falls on general tax revenue. The national and regional Governments together contribute more than eighty percent. The premiums and matching employers' payments represent about eleven percent. Patients paying a portion of their bills cover about six percent of the costs.

Despite the long Swedish tradition of solo practice, hospital and group practice are now on the upswing. Organized medicine has ended its long battle against the national health system, and has learned that the most effective way to influence it is from the inside. Doctors, who are now prominent on the twenty-eight regional health insurance boards, cooperate in planning, organization, and administration.

Dr. Arne Ekengren, vice-president of the Swedish Medical Association, told an interviewer from *Medical Economics*, "Most doctors and virtually the entire population are now happy with the national health insurance program. . . . We Swedes can be stubborn at times, and that includes physicians. However, we are not unreasonable people, and, after a while, we began to see the reason for national health insurance. For example, one of the arguments against the program was that two-thirds of the population was covered by voluntary health insurance. However, we now know that the people who really needed full health coverage—the poor and the people on the economic borderline between the poor and the fairly well-off—didn't get it. Today they do."

While there are other factors involved, it should be noted that Sweden leads the list of nations in life expectancy at birth for males, is second on the list in life expectancy at birth for females, and is lowest in infant mortality.

The German Way

Germany was the pioneer in national health insurance and, like other pioneers in uncharted terrains, made some frightful mistakes. These mistakes set the stage for horrendous struggles with the medical profession. Today, the West German system is the most flexible, the least centralized, and involves the least government intervention.

When Bismarck instituted a national health system in 1883, he did not have to worry much about the doctors, who had not yet organized, so he wrote a plan that put power primarily in the hands of the sick funds, which could engage restricted panels of physicians, set their fees, and bar the rest from insurance practice. He *did* have to worry about business interests, which successfully opposed a higher tax on employers than on employees. Since, unlike the health plans in other countries, the German plan also provided for no Government contribution at all, the result was chronic under-financing, and the result of *that* was a squeeze on the underpaid doctors.

It has taken seventy years of organization, agitation, law suits, and strikes for the German medical profession to undo some of the handicaps that Bismarck put on them. It was not until 1955 that the insurance doctors got rid of their status as employees of the sick funds and became instead the contract administrators. It was not until 1960 that a court decision declared it unconstitutional to bar a doctor from insurance practice. Today eighty-five percent of the doctors have insurance practice, though they are also free to practice privately.

Today, eighty-five percent of the West German population is covered by a system that is compulsory for all workers whose income falls below a certain minimum, most pensioners, and many self-employed persons. The well-to-do take care of themselves, and the unemployed rely on charity. The system is administered through some 2,000 sick funds, organized by locality or by factory. (There are also sixteen special funds which offer greater benefits for those who want to travel first-class by paying higher contributions.) Employers and employees share the premiums equally.

The centerpiece of the German system is the *Krankenschein*, or "sickness ticket." The beneficiary gets the *Krankenschein* from his employer or local sick fund, presents it to his doctor, who records on it the treatment given and sends it to the

Insurance Doctors' Association for reimbursement. The patient is free to choose his doctor, and the doctor may not make any charge to the patient (except when the patient insists on some procedure which the doctor considers medically unnecessary and therefore unchargeable to insurance). Drugs are free, except for a nominal charge per prescription to discourage over-utilization.

It is thus a fee-for-service system, based on an incredibly voluminous schedule of fees for specific services. (It includes, for example, what the doctor may charge for a telephone conversation with his patient.) The role of the Government is to establish the minimum coverage, the maximum premiums (currently eleven percent of wages), and maximum fees. The rest is basically left to negotiation between the insurance doctors and the insurance funds. This system, in which the doctors' association itself handles the distribution of the money and sets individual fees after negotiating lump-sum contracts with the insurance funds, is unique.

With fees generally on the low side, the doctor has an incentive to multiply procedures and compete for sickness tickets in order to maintain his income. To win popularity, some doctors are lenient about certifying workers for sickness benefits, which may help to account for West Germany's unusually high rate of disability payment. On the other hand, the doctors have an incentive to police their own colleagues because they are all sharing a lump sum negotiated with the insurance fund and limited by the government ceiling on premiums.

West Germany's health-care program, unlike that of Sweden, is concentrated on the doctor's office. There is little competition from hospital outpatient departments. Hospital doctors may see insurance cases during their off hours in the hospital, but only when referred by the private practitioner. A West German's insurance covers an unlimited stay in the hospital, which is generally run by the local government and has its own staff of salaried physicians.

The insurance system is generally popular in West Germany. An opinion survey indicated that ninety percent of beneficiaries would continue if it were made voluntary. Also, in 1965, when upper-bracket employees were allowed to opt out by joining a voluntary plan, only two percent of them chose to do so.

That is not to say that the German system has not shown some weaknesses. One is the competitive element that has resulted in what insurance administrators call "the patient-hunting doctor." Another weakness is the tendency toward wasteful duplication of services. One study showed that the smaller a doctor's case load, the greater his average number of services per patient. Like the United States, West Germany suffers from a maldistribution of doctors since physicians tend to cluster in large industrial cities where there are more sickness tickets to be collected.

In Europe no country with national health insurance considers its system ideal. Each is still tinkering with it, trying to get rid of the bugs. None could conceive of abolishing it for, by and large, the comprehensive systems have opened the doors of health to millions to whom they were closed before.

CHAPTER X

THE DRIVE FOR NATIONAL HEALTH INSURANCE

The year 1970 could be noted in history as the year national health insurance got off the ground. It will certainly be remembered as the year that it became a serious public issue.

Through most of this century public health has been kicked around as an idea. Occasionally it has surfaced for discussion, only to submerge again under the weight of apathy and barrages against any structural changes, the American Medical Association labeling it as "Socialism and Communism—inciting to revolution."

Since 1934 there have been official proposals—first by the Roosevelt Administration, later by the Truman Administration. Its advocates, at various times, included Senators Robert F. Wagner, Robert Taft, Jacob Javits, Governor Earl Warren of California, and Representative Richard M. Nixon of California (who, as presidential candidate in 1968, campaigned against the idea, saying, "New health programs should be geared only to persons in need").

Since 1943, starting with the Wagner-Murray-Dingell bill, there have been recommendations recurrently dropped into the overstuffed Congressional hoppers to die unsung with each session of Congress.

The 1965 enactment of Medicare, for the first time recognizing 20 million aging Americans as entitled to public health protection, was regarded by many as the opening of the door to a more comprehensive plan. Others, however, hoped that by "settling" the problem of the most vulnerable, Medicare might, in fact, ease the pressure for national health insurance.

In 1970, as the average American gasped at the dizzying spiral of health costs, a national health plan gave signs of turning from a minority into a majority issue. It emerged from the conference room to the public stump, generated a cluster of bills and a series of Congressional hearings, and attracted the interest of politicians as a promising election issue.

Our neighbors on this continent and in Europe could smile in tolerant perplexity that we were now agonizing over what they had long ago settled. Germany has had a health insurance law since the time of Chancellor Bismarck in the 1880s.

Since then every important western nation has gone on to adopt one—most recently Canada in 1968. Two European countries—the Soviet Union and Great Britain—have gone beyond national health *insurance* to develop national health *services.*

If this is now to be an issue in a great debate, it may be well to clarify the distinction between national health *insurance* and National Health *Services,* which has been a source of considerable confusion, not all of it unintentional. National health *insurance* is a government-subsidized system of paying health bills. A National Health *Service* provides the treatment and, in so doing, employs or at least sets the working conditions for the medical personnel. That emotion-laden phrase, "socialized medicine," to the extent that it means anything, can only be properly applied to the latter.

It may surprise many to know that we already have quite a bit of "socialized medicine." Wilbur Cohen, former secretary of HEW, figures "socialized medicine" at about $6 billion worth annually, or ten percent of the nation's health expenditures. That includes $3 billion in medical services for the armed forces and veterans, plus hospitalization for the tuberculous, the mentally ill, the mentally retarded, and medical services for Indians. Uncle Sam, the doctor, is an easily accepted figure where special groups who do not raise emotional or ideological problems are involved.

Health *insurance* under Government auspices dates back to 1798, when Congress provided a contributory hospital scheme for merchant seamen. The big advance in public insurance coverage came, of course, with Medicare. The Johnson Administration proposed extending Medicare protection to the disabled, but there has been no action so far because of Congressional worries about mounting costs.

The next idea for extending coverage came from the Nixon Administration. Groping for an exit from the inequities and iniquities of Medicaid, it proposed a new health insurance scheme for 5 to 6 million poor families with children—the ones to be covered by its Family Assistance Program. It proposed to provide a $500 premium-value policy to cover a package of hospital, outpatient, and preventive services. It would be compulsory in certain categories. While the most destitute would get it free, others would have to pay a percentage of their incomes in premiums.

Thus, the Nixon Administration proposed to introduce the first health insurance in the nation's history that, for some at least, would be both compulsory and subject to a personal fee.

Medicare hospital insurance is compulsory and supported by a tax, but that tax is not on the individual. It is spread, through Social Security, among the nation's working people, paid in their productive years when they can best afford it. Medicare's doctor insurance requires the individual to contribute, but it is optional. Thus, the Nixon Administration's proposal, while representing movement toward expansion of health insurance coverage, also displayed backward movement in singling out the poor as the subjects of the first direct, forced tax for health—to be deducted from their welfare payments.

This proposal only underlined the broader issue—whether the time has come to replace piecemeal protection by a system of comprehensive and universal health insurance for all Americans.

The Nixon Administration had been inclined to shun anything so ambitious. It was jolted when the National Governors' Conference, thirty of them Republicans, adopted a resolution in Colorado Springs in September, 1969, urging adoption of a national health insurance program. Then HEW Secretary Robert Finch suddenly amended his mandate to Walter McNerney's Task Force on Medicaid and Related Problems, asking it to consider "long-term methods of financing the nation's medical care."

Word was later passed to the task force that the Administration did not want to see a national health insurance plan emerge. So the task force reported that it was not "the appropriate body" to develop such a plan. But it did put the issue up to the Administration by saying:

"It seems to us vital that the Department develop a policy

position on this critical and controversial health-care issue. Such policy is necessary as a measure against which to appraise the proposals which Congress will soon be considering. It also seems to us necessary that the Department assume the initiative on an issue so central to its responsibilities. ... Since next steps may well set public and private patterns for at least a decade, the nation ought not to proceed in so large and grave a policy area without fully informed debate."

The task force urged the appointment of "a high-level body" to study a national health-care financing policy and have recommendations ready for the 1971 session of Congress. It suggested guidelines for the study, including the following:

1. No individual shall be deprived of needed health care because of inability to pay. . . . No one should be encouraged to delay care because of an insurance system that will not pay for ambulatory or preventive care. . . .

2. No family should suffer substantial hardship because of the expenses of unpredictable illness or accident. . . . A national policy should not have limits that make the costs of health care a substantial burden for an individual or family.

3. The financing method should make the level of public spending on health responsive to . . . public preferences. It should neither freeze expenditures at current levels nor lead to excessive future investment in health services.

4. A financing system should wield incentives to maximize efficiency and effective use of resources and to discourage health-care price inflation. . . . Therefore, the financing method should encourage cost-consciousness in the decisions of patients, doctors, and hospital administrators.

5. The administration of a health-care system should not require complex procedures or encourage arbitrary decisions of patients. . . . Capitation and direct private payment are administratively simpler than individual reimbursement of customary charges or costs. . . .

6. Any method of financing should be acceptable to the general public and to health-care personnel and institutions.

This challenge from its task force and the awareness of things in motion outside the Administration put a department which had been trying to duck the issue of national health insurance as premature on an uncomfortable spot. The department's position had been, as Undersecretary John Veneman put it in an interview with me, "We have to restructure the health delivery system, and then get a more effective way of making the payments for the services that are provided. All that health insurance would do now would be to provide a different mechanism to pay the bills that we are now getting."

Dr. James Cavanaugh, Deputy Assistant Secretary for Health, had stated it even more strongly. "National health insurance will only spread the financial risk of illness. It will have no impact, in and by itself, on reducing cost but rather would immediately increase cost. . . . This approach, in and by itself, will do little more than perpetuate an inefficient health system that is already to the point of collapse."

There were, indeed, some in the administration who, without wishing to be quoted publicly, were expressing dark suspicions that some of the advocates of national insurance were hoping to create a situation of confrontation and breakdown that would lead to complete socialization of health services. Outside the Administration, taking a less conspirational view, were analysts like Dr. Charles Lewis of Harvard, who also feared the effect of early broadening of insurance coverage.

"Given the current system of delivering care, fee-for-service, essentially in non-group or small-group practices, the costs would escalate, and they would escalate extremely rapidly," he said. "As costs escalate out of sight, the consumer, I think, would demand control either of costs or, more likely, of the whole system. . . . If we were unable to deliver, except at enormous costs, I think frustration would go very rapidly right through the ceiling. I'm not for that kind of confrontation."

The American Hospital Association had a similar warning. In an interview Dr. Mark Berke, American Hospital Association president, said, "I think that if we simply talk about the financing of health care and making it easier for the public to get the necessary health care, and we simply pour billions of dollars into this funnel, we're simply going to force prices up. We're not going to provide much more care. History has shown this in the Medicare program. We poured billions of dollars into health care, the prices boomed up, and yet the figures do not show that there has been any major increase in the amount of medical care given to the public in the United States. . . . We have to make some changes in the availability, the accessibility, and the organization and delivery of health care."

The American Medical Association took the stand that quality of patient care would suffer if health insurance were broadened too soon. I asked Dr. Gerald Dorman, president, what would happen if Congress were to enact a universal health insurance system now.

"I think the doctors would be more than busy," said Dr. Dorman. "They might even be killing themselves with overwork. I think that it would be financially a bonanza to have everybody coming in. I don't think we have enough doctors to take care of the people who would come. There would be a gradual crescendo of patients who would almost swamp us before we could get our facilities up to the point where we could take care of it.

"In such a landslide of business, the tendency, very often, is not to give enough time to each patient. . . . I'm not against this idea of covering us all. We're all working for it. But give us a little time to catch up to it. And there isn't a system for doing it."

But this view presupposed that national health insurance, like Medicare, would simply pour in money without incentives and controls. Enough has been learned from the Medicare experience to suggest that a comprehensive insurance law

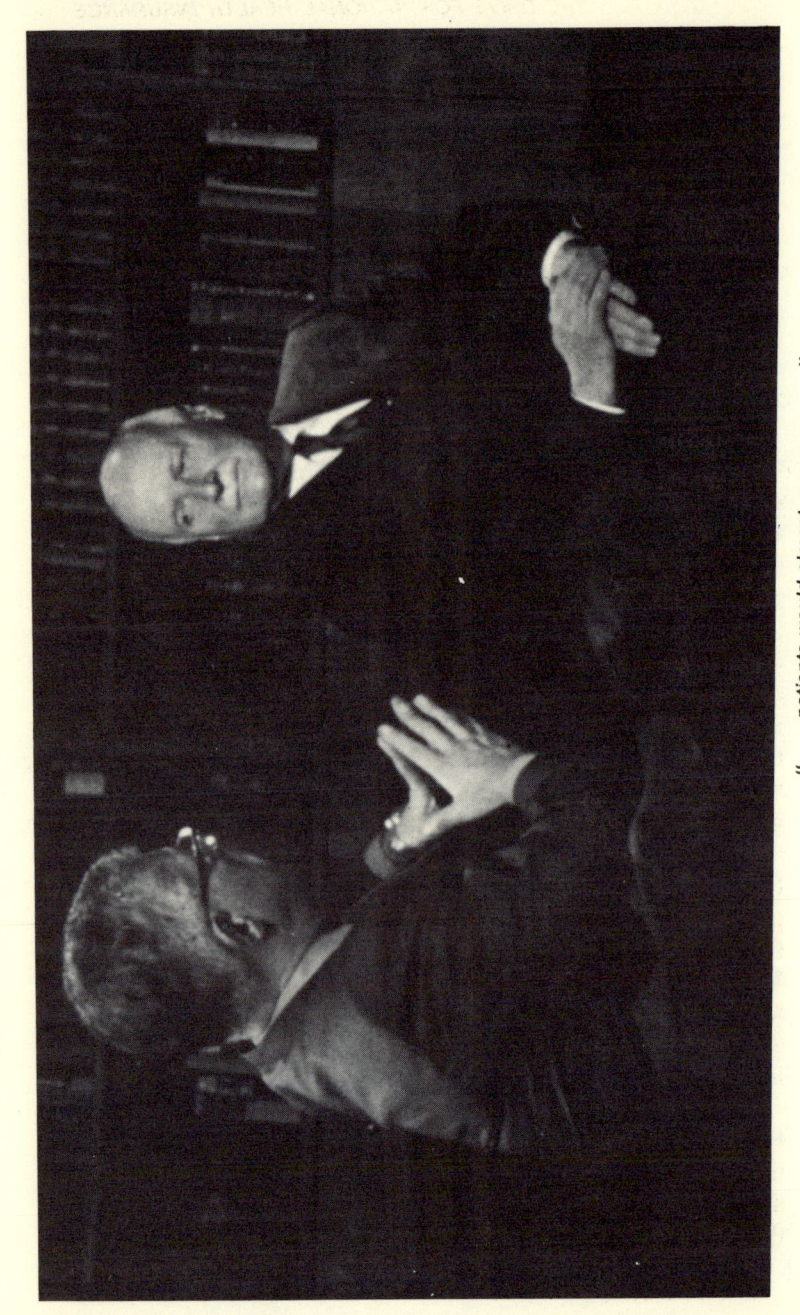

"... patients would almost swamp us ..."

could avoid some of these pitfalls, as the McNerney task force has stressed it would have to. Against the argument for delay was the argument for speed made by activists like Dr. Rashi Fein:

"National health insurance, an expression of the right to medical care, will necessitate that somebody assume responsibility and, in assuming responsibility, will have to help to create a better system. We have learned from experience—from the prepaid group practice plans, from the neighborhood health centers—that we can provide health care for a population on an organized basis.

"There are those who say 'why not prepare?' I do not think that if we set 1980 as the date for a national health insurance system, we would spend the decade of the seventies preparing. I would guess that we would wake up on December 31, 1979, saying, 'Oh my gosh! We have only one day left! We had better get down to work!'

"I think that supply responds to demand. There *would* be a problem of people trying to go to doctors and not finding doctors available. That would bring out into the open what is now happening. Today, there are people who don't go to the doctor because we have rationed them out of the market by price. We charge high enough prices so that they don't go. I'd rather have this out in the open.

"I think that it's healthier to have the queues, to have people frustrated, so that we see that there are people who are not getting medical care because of a shortage of physicians, or because of lack of organization. I don't want to cover it up. We could eliminate our problems tomorrow by charging $1,000 for a physician's visit. You and I would stay home when we got sick. That's not the way to solve the problem. . . .

"If we institute a national health insurance system, there will be strains, there will be pressures. But I do not think that the American system will legislate changes first, and I am willing to push for national insurance because I think that this will force us to address the problem of change.

"You may think that this is a dangerous philosophy to

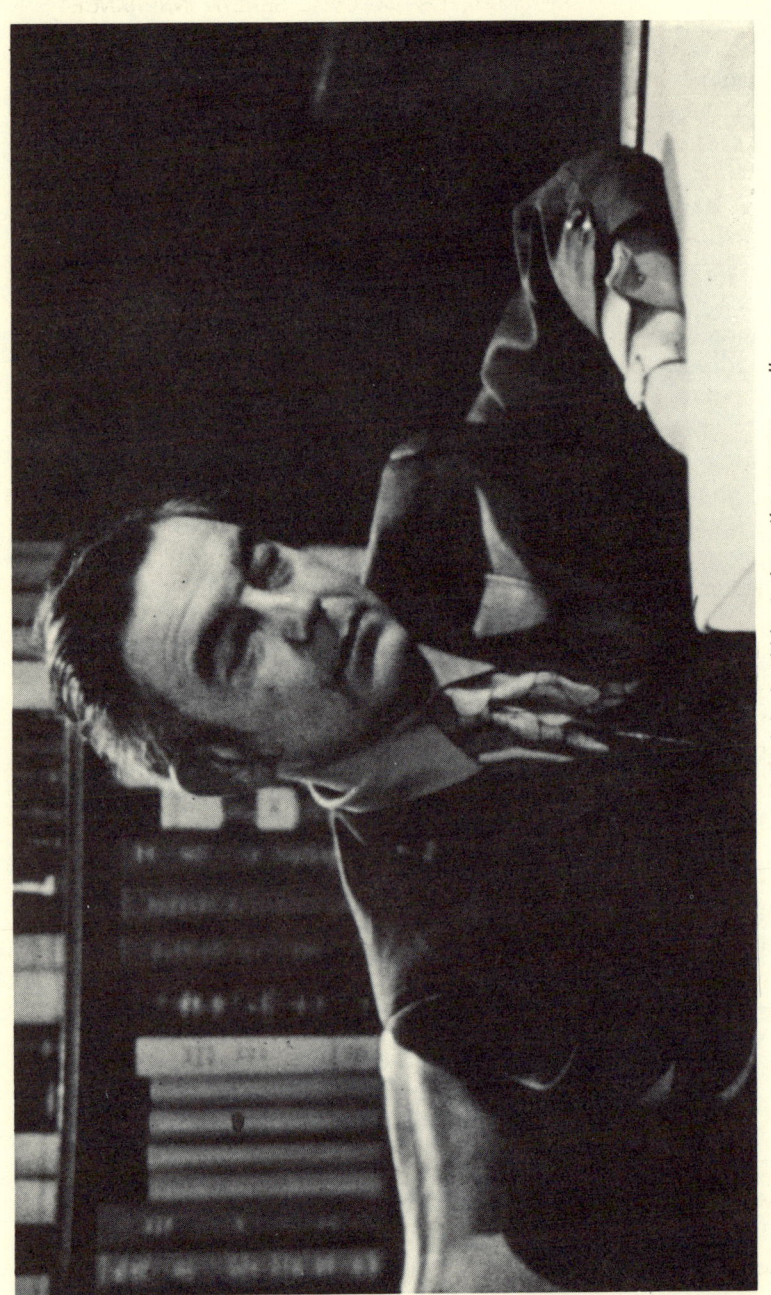

"I think its healthier to have the queues. . . ."

counsel. But, in fact, we have learned from Medicare and Medicaid, and the Administration's current policies in those programs suggest that in the enactment of national health insurance we would be more careful than we were.

"We would be able to do things that we weren't able to do in the past. We would be willing to intervene where we wanted to step aside in the past. So I don't think that we are really likely to enact a national health insurance program that doesn't provide the proper incentives. And, to the extent that we fall short, I think that we would correct it in a year."

The remarkable fact is that few in authority still argue against the principle of national health insurance. They argue about whether the egg or the chicken should come first— whether an insurance system should await a necessary change in the delivery system, or whether the insurance system should be instituted, hoping to force that change. In 1970, the longstanding controversy had changed from pro-anti to a controversy about how broad an insurance system, with how much intervention into the delivery of medical services, and to be started when?

To avoid having to deal with issues like these, President Nixon postponed plans for a message on health, leaving a conspicuous gap in his series of messages on national problems in his first eighteen months in office.

The new HEW secretary, Elliot Richardson, who had not immediately reacted to the urging of the McNerney task force to develop a national health-care financing policy, said in an interview, that his priority was improving the present system and, if this could be done, pressure for national health insurance could be contained.

"I don't think I could predict at this stage that it will come," he said. "It may come, whether or not it does is certainly going to depend in considerable measure on the success with which we can contain costs and improve the delivery, availability, and quality of medical care for the people who are getting it now.

"A national health program would, in effect, extend health insurance to a lot of people who are getting good medical care now and who are able to pay for it. So the question is: What do you have to do to make sure that those who aren't getting it, who aren't able to pay for it, do get it and are assisted in paying for it?"

Mr. Richardson disagreed with those who contend that national insurance is needed to get the leverage to improve the delivery of health care. "What is more urgent is the development of techniques, devices, and an organizational system that can improve delivery and quality of care. And if we knew how to do that, then I think we would find that we have the leverage already without moving down the road to a national health insurance system."

So, with the Administration apparently unwilling to join in formulating a program, the early stage of the debate was pre-empted by a widely varying series of proposals that came to Congress from groups with special concerns.

There are five national health insurance schemes under discussion. They can be roughly grouped as two social insurance or Government-operated plans, two private insurance plans, and one that represents a compromise between the public and the private approach.

Here is how they look, in general terms, reading from "left to right," or from most liberal to most conservative:

1. The Reuther Plan.

This plan was developed by the Committee for National Health Insurance, also known as "The Committee of One Hundred," headed by the late Walter Reuther, president of the United Auto Workers. It is sponsored in Congress by three senators who are members of that committee—Edward M. Kennedy of Massachusetts and Ralph W. Yarborough of Texas, Democrats, and John Sherman Cooper of Kentucky, Republican. Twelve other senators have joined them.

It provides for a program covering all residents of the United States, administered by a five-man Health Security Board named by the President and serving in the Department of HEW. It would be financed by a tax on payroll and non-earned income and by general Federal revenues.

Its comprehensive benefits would cover almost everything generally recognized as health services. There would be limitations on coverage of mental health services, skilled nursing home services, dental care, drugs, and appliances.

Under the Health Security Board, regional and local offices would be given strong discretionary powers to provide flexibility. The board would be counseled by a Health Security Advisory Council, whose majority would consist of consumer representatives.

All providers would receive payments on the basis of budgets intended to pay reasonable cost under efficient operation. There would be emphasis on expansion of preventive health care and early diagnosis of illness. Financial and other incentives would be provided to physicians to form new medical care groups and teams. A special fund would be used to help the expansion of group medical practice. Duplicating services would be gradually eliminated by withdrawal of funding. Priority would be given, in payment of physicians, to those on salary and in prepaid group practice.

The estimated cost of the program, if it had gone into effect in 1969, is $37 billion, including $6 billion in new Federal expenditures.

2. The Griffiths (AFL-CIO) Plan.

This plan, which the AFL-CIO helped to develop, was introduced in the House of Representatives in February, 1970, by Representative Martha Griffiths, Democrat, of Michigan. In many respects it resembles the Reuther Plan, but is somewhat less far-reaching.

More types of benefits would be subject to limitations, and for some the cost would be shared by the patient (co-payment), up to an annual maximum of $50 a person or $100 for a family.

It would be administered by a nine-member National Health Insurance Board, headed by the Secretary of HEW, with two other Government representatives, plus representation from labor, employers, providers of care, and medical-care and administrative specialists. Two advisory councils would represent the health professions and consumers. Regional administrators would be responsible for contracting with providers of care and dealing with complaints, quality of care, and manpower problems.

Organized groups of physicians could contract to provide service, receiving payment on a negotiated budget (capitation) basis. Individual physicians could also arrange to be paid on a capitation basis. (There appears to be less pressure than in the Reuther plan to form group practices.) Hospitals would be paid on a negotiated budget or other approved basis.

The cost of the program, if it had gone into effect in 1969, is estimated by the AFL-CIO at $35.8 billion.

There are indications that the Reuther plan and the Griffiths plan will be merged. Leonard Woodcock, Reuther's successor as president of the United Auto Workers, has met with George Meany, president of the AFL-CIO, and they have agreed to work for a joint health insurance plan.

3. The Javits Bill

This plan, introduced in the Senate in April, 1970, by Jacob Javits, Republican, of New York, represents a compromise between social and private insurance. It is based on an expansion of the Medicare program, with an option to "elect out" of the Government program by the purchase of approved private insurance.

Under its terms, the Medicare program would be extended to the disabled in July, 1971, and at the same time the voluntary doctor's coverage in that program would be merged with the compulsory hospital insurance. Starting in July, 1973, it would be extended to the general population. Benefits, far more restricted than in the preceding two plans, would be the same as in the current Medicare program, with additional ones to be added later.

The Department of HEW would have responsibility for administration, as under the present Medicare program. By agreement with HEW, state governments could accept responsibility for administering all or part of the program. As under Medicare, private insurance companies would process the benefit claims under contract with HEW. Under certain conditions, however, the Secretary of HEW could establish a public corporation to handle claims in certain areas.

Payment to providers of service would be under current conditions of "reasonable costs" for hospitals and "reasonable charges" for physicians until June, 1973, when a new reimbursement procedure would be instituted, designed to control cost and utilization and improve the organization of medical services, but assuring providers of fair and reasonable compensation. The plan includes incentives for efficiency in the form of a sharing in savings produced by health-care service systems.

The program would be financed by a payroll tax for employers and employees, a parallel tax for the self-employed, and an equal contribution by the Federal Government. The Social Security Administration (whose analysis was invaluable in compiling this summary of the plans) estimates the cost of the program at $22.7 billion in 1975.

4. The Pettengill Proposal.

This is a private, as opposed to social, insurance plan. It was drafted by Daniel W. Pettengill, vice-president of Aetna Life and Casualty Company, the most active commercial company in the health insurance field. It was presented to the House Ways and Means Committee in November, 1969, and is basically aimed at supplementing Medicare and replacing Medicaid.

It would provide special health insurance for the poor, near-poor, and high-risk "uninsurable" persons through an insurance pool administered by private companies, partly financed by Federal and state funds. Its coverage would be limited to persons not already covered by Medicare. Participation would be voluntary, but the states would be required to cover their welfare recipients.

Each state would establish a uniform health insurance plan, but would be required to meet minimum Federal standards.

COMPARISON OF FIVE PROPOSALS FOR NATIONAL HEALTH INSURANCE[1]

PROPOSALS	GENERAL APPROACH	COVERAGE	BENEFITS
Griffiths Bill	Government universal health insurance program financed by payroll tax and general revenues.	U.S. residents	Comprehensive health benefits. Major exclusion is dental services for adults. No cost-sharing except for physician, dentist, and other ambulatory services. ($2 co-pay per visit, with certain exceptions.)
Committee for National Health Insurance	Government universal health insurance program financed by payroll tax and general revenues.	U.S. residents	Comprehensive health benefits. Major exclusion is dental services for adults. Limitations on podiatrists' services, drugs, nursing home, and mental health care. No cost-sharing.
Javits Bill	Government universal health insurance program (similar to Medicare) with option of "electing out" by purchase of private insurance.[2]	U.S. residents	Same as Medicare (hospital, physician, nursing home, etc.—subject to cost-sharing and limitations). Also, annual check-ups, limited drugs, and dental care for children under age eight.
AMA Medicredit	Income tax credits to offset cost of qualified private health insurance.[3]	U.S. residents (voluntary).	To be qualified, policy must include basic hospital and physician benefits, and may optionally offer supplementary drug, blood, hospital and other benefits. Benefits subject generally to cost-sharing and limitations.
Pettengill Proposal	Private insurance for poor or related groups through an insurance pool subsidized by government.[4]	Poor, near poor, and uninsurables (voluntary).	Statewide uniform benefits. Minimum benefits to be specified in Federal law and to include ambulatory and institutional care.

COMPARISON OF FIVE PROPOSALS (CON'T)

PROPOSALS	ADMINISTRATION	PAYMENT OF PROVIDERS
Griffiths Bill	Federal board composed of HEW officials and nongovernment members; regional offices; advisory bodies.	Physician and dentist groups can contract to receive pre-determined payment and pay their members as they choose (including fee for service). Individual primary physicians and dentists may elect per capita, salary, or combination of methods and receive an allowance to pay for services of specialists and other health professionals. Hospitals: Negotiated budget that includes allowance for nursing home and home health services.
Committee for National Health Insurance	Federal board under Department of HEW; regional offices; advisory bodies.	Physicians and dentists: Regional funds allocated first to those in group practice or selecting capitation, salary, or per session basis. Residual allocated to local payment authorities to pay those selecting fee-for-service or per case basis. Hospitals, nursing homes, home health agencies: Negotiated budget designed to pay reasonable cost under efficient organization.
Javits Bill	Department of HEW (as under Medicare) or, under contract with HEW, by state government. Processing of claims conducted by private carriers (as under Medicare) or, under certain conditions, by special quasi-government organizations.	Until July 1, 1973, reasonable cost for hospital and institutions and reasonable charges for physicians (as under Medicare). Thereafter, new methods, developed in interim, may be employed.
AMA Medicredit	Federal advisory board (including HEW, IRS, and nongovernment members) to establish federal standards for use by state insurance departments in approving private insurance plans.	Present methods under private insurance.
Pettengill Proposal	Statewide insurance pool administered by carrier selected by state with concurrence of federal government.	Present methods under private insurance.

COMPARISON OF FIVE PROPOSALS (CON'T)

PROPOSALS	FINANCING	COST
Griffiths Bill	Tax equal to 7 percent of payroll, including 1 percent on employees, 3 percent on employers, and a payment from general revenues equal to 3 percent. Earnings base of $15,000, adjusted automatically to increases in wage levels.	Cost would have been $35.8 billion in fiscal 1969, according to AFL-CIO.
Committee for National Health Insurance	Tax equal to about 7¾ percent (on 1969 basis) including 2.8 percent on employers, 1.8 percent on employees and on nonwage income, and general revenues payment equal to 3.1 percent. Tax levied on first $15,000 of employees and nonwage income combined, and on total payroll per employers.	Cost would have been $37 billion in fiscal 1969, according to CNHI.
Javits Bill	Tax equal to 10 percent of payroll, including 3.3 percent on employers and 3.3 percent on employees and payment from general revenues equal to 3.3 percent. Tax levied on $15,000 earnings base for employees and on total payroll for employers.	Cost of $22.7 billion in 1975, according to Social Security actuary.
AMA Medicredit	Financed from federal general revenues	Net cost for 1970 estimated at $8 billion by AMA and at $15 billion by SSA
Pettengill Proposal	Poor would pay no premium and the near poor and uninsurables would pay part of the premium. State and federal general revenues would finance the balance of the cost of the program.	Estimates not available.

[1] Source: Social Security Administration.
[2] Participants in approved employer-employee health plans and persons purchasing approved private insurance may remain outside of government plan and be exempted from payroll taxes.
[3] Amount of tax credit would be graduated from 100 percent to 10 percent, depending on the amount of tax liability on tax returns. The maximum (100 percent) credit would be an amount equal to the premium cost of a qualified health insurance policy.
[4] Other provisions of this plan are designed to improve insurance coverage for the working population.

It would be administered through an insurance pool, supervised by the state insurance agency, with all carriers participating. There would be no change in present methods of reimbursing providers of medical services.

The poor would pay no premium, the near-poor would pay part of their premium, the uninsurable would pay a rate which, to some extent, would reflect their high claims cost. The premiums would be paid into a pool, which would not be enough to cover the benefits. The deficit would be shared by state and Federal Governments.

There is no estimate of what the public cost of this program would be.

5. The Medicredit Plan.

This proposal, sponsored by the American Medical Association, was outlined to the House Ways and Means Committee in November, 1969, and its concept is embodied in a bill introduced by Richard Fulton, Democrat, of Tennessee and Senator Paul Fannin, Republican, of Arizona.

It would leave Medicare untouched, but would replace Medicaid for all poor and near-poor persons under sixty-five. It would provide tax credits to offset the premium cost of private health insurance purchased voluntarily. The scale of credits would be graduated, depending on income.

Under the Fulton-Fannin bill, a family earning $5,000 or less would receive a one hundred percent tax credit on Federal income up to $400. If a family were liable for less than $400 in taxes, the Government would issue a voucher to make up the difference.

The American Medical Association's version differs principally in that it reckons tax liability rather than income and in that it does not set a maximum credit, but says the maximum would be determined by the premium cost of a "qualified" health insurance policy. Such a policy would have to include sixty days of hospital inpatient care, subject to an annual $50 deductible; hospital and outpatient care, subject to twenty percent co-insurance up to a $100 maximum in co-insurance, and physician's services on the same basis. The deductible and co-insurance would be waived for those entitled to the maximum tax credit, that is, those with a tax liability less than $300.

The program would be administered by a Health Insurance Advisory Board, headed by the secretary of HEW.

The American Medical Association estimates that the total cost of the plan in 1970 would have been $14.6 billion, and the net cost $8.3 billion, after making allowance for savings in Medicaid and the number of persons who would presumably not avail themselves of the plan. The Social Security Administration figures $15.3 billion, a more realistic estimate of the net cost.

In its original form, the American Medical Association left the delivery of services virtually unmentioned. A belated revision provided for review of utilization, charges, and quality of services rendered by providers. It also provided that disciplinary action, including suspension or exclusion from the program, could be imposed under specified procedures.

There is thus a spectrum of plans, all called national health insurance, all claiming to answer the question: How do we provide adequate medical service to those who are not getting it?

The conservative plans suggest that some more money dropped in the right place will do it. The liberal plans are based on the premise that it cannot be done without a fundamental overhaul of America's health system.

The opponents of the conservative plans see perils in pouring more money into a system that is not working. The opponents of the liberal plans see perils in Government control, worry about a medical profession in chains, and perceive socialism at the end of the road.

There is a growing consensus that the time is long overdue for this nation to have a national plan for health.

"I think," said Mark Berke, "that this country is going to have some sort of universal health insurance coverage for everybody in the United States."

"I think," said Walter McNerney, "of a system in which

THE DRIVE FOR NATIONAL HEALTH INSURANCE

the Federal Government plays a very active role in setting standards and supplying money—a more sophisticated role for the entire population."

"A better system," said Dr. Rashi Fein, "will only be created when the American public is ready, willing, and able to work towards that end, and the prime requirement is that it understand."

"I would imagine," said Dr. Gerald Dorman, "that it would be another five or ten years before we're ready for it, but this could be taken in steps."

"I think," said Dr. Charles Lewis, "that it is undoubtedly necessary to escalate the conflict to the point at which the alternative becomes absolutely essential. I see it as a sort of Cuban missile crisis for the medical profession."

Dr. Lewis was suggesting, as many others have, that the principal barrier to a national health insurance system is organized medicine and its powerful lobby in Washington, and that its resistance will only be overcome if—like Nikita Khrushchev in Cuba—it is brought eyeball to eyeball with a prospect more menacing to its position.

"In fact," said Wilbur Cohen, "health insurance has become the bulwark against socialized medicine."

Clearly, the health professions cannot be dragooned into a new health-care system. It cannot be done, said Walter McNerney, "if there is simply sullen compliance." But the monolith of organized medicine has shown signs of bending, and there is a more flexible spirit in the ranks of the doctors. Forty-eight percent of physicians are no longer dues-paying members of the American Medical Association.

"I think," said Dr. Fein, "that organized medicine will be taken on, and I think that we will establish civilian control over the health sector, as we have established civilian control over the military."

Now, when even the American Medical Association finds it necessary to have its own horse, however spavined, entered in the national health insurance derby, it seems clear that the starter's gun has been heard and the race is on. It will be a grueling race—far more grueling than the Medicare

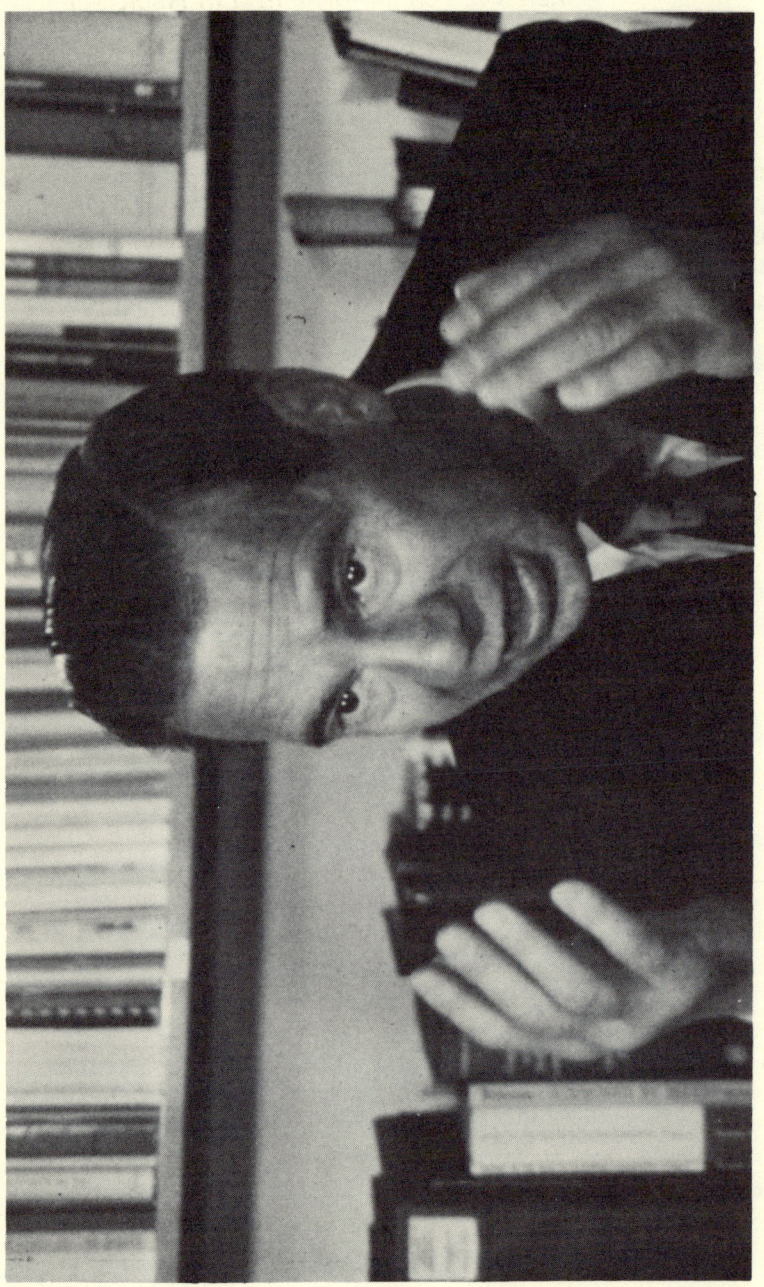

"... this country is going to have some sort of universal health insurance coverage...."

contest, which was, in effect, a preliminary to this national controversy.

It may go on for years—efforts to put band-aids on the present system, with cost-control decrees and new arrangements for the poor, while the campaign for national health insurance gathers force. But the signs are that before too long the United States will join the rest of the civilized world in accepting the "right to health" and in making it a reality.

APPENDIX ONE

The Task Force on Medicaid and Related programs, with Walter J. McNerney, president of the Blue Cross Association, as chairman, had twenty-seven members representing the viewpoints of consumers, industry, labor, Government, and the social sciences, as well as the medical profession and health institutions and services. This is the introduction and summary of recommendations of this task force, as submitted to Elliot Richardson, Secretary of HEW, on June 29, 1970.

INTRODUCTION

The task force was requested by the Secretary of Health, Education, and Welfare, in July 1969, to examine the deficiencies of Medicaid[1] and related programs and to make recommendations for improvement within the context of existing legislation and with regard to the need for new legislation. Subsequently, in September 1969, the charge was broadened to include considerations involved in long-term methods of financing the nation's medical care.

During its deliberations, the task force was aware of the rising public concern with the cost and availability of health services, a concern that has emerged on occasion in the language used to describe the health system as "in a crisis," "badly fragmented," and "in serious trouble." Members of the task force are also aware that the problems—whether of policy or system, managerial or professional, racial or social—are deep-seated and that their successful resolution will tax the ingenuity and resources of the public and private sectors.

---

[1] Enacted in 1965, title XIX of the Social Security Act established Medicaid, a federal-state medical public assistance program which, at the option of the states, makes vendor payments to providers of medical services on behalf of recipients of cash maintenance payments and on behalf of other categories of people (the "medically indigent") who need help in meeting medical expenses.

The system is large—currently more than $60 billion a year is being spent on health. In terms of ownership and programs the health system is also complex and variegated. The spate of legislative and scientific changes introduced in the last decade, with the best of intentions, has not been easily or consistently incorporated. One regrettable result is that there is fairly widespread cynicism about oversold promises that must be taken into account. The road ahead will not be easy; effective intervention will require heroic and sophisticated measures to match the size and complexity of the problems.

As the task force grappled with its charges, several themes emerged that merit recognition in setting the stage for recommendations. One that was expressed repeatedly during the discussions was the conviction that health must remain high on the scale of social, economic, and political priorities—not only because the health of the nation is basic to the growth and productivity of the economy but also because human compassion insists that essential individual health needs shall be met.

With rapidly rising costs, many misgivings were expressed about the growing tendency to become excessively preoccupied with cost at the expense of community goals. The task force, along with what is possibly a majority in the health professions and certainly a majority of the population, considers the recent Federal enactments as intending that access to basic medical care shall be a right or entitlement of all citizens. It is the position of the task force that the right or entitlement is not fulfilled when millions in the population do not know about or cannot get to the places where some care is available to deprived populations, or when the millions who do get to such places are given a kind of service that is woefully inferior by every standard known to man and doctor. Neither is the right or entitlement concept honored just because physicians and hospital administrators can say, "We never turn away a patient." However virtuous the declaration may make the doctors and hospital people feel, it does nothing to make good the right or entitlement for those who never get within sight of a doctor's office or hospital.

APPENDIX ONE

The promise of Medicaid that some care, at least, would be available to all who needed it has vanished into the obscurity of state determinations of eligibility and the parsimony of state determinations of solvency. How completely the promise vanished is suggested by the task force estimate that only about one-third of the 30 to 40 million indigent and medically indigent who could potentially be covered by title XIX of the Social Security Act will, in fact, receive services. That the cost of covering less than one-third has exceeded earlier estimates of the cost of covering the whole medically deprived population is due to a combination of factors, including inflation. It also suggests how badly the expenditures have been controlled or how badly the program costs were estimated or both.

The Medicaid recommendations presented here are directed not only toward correcting the most obvious inequities of Medicaid coverage by establishing a "Federal floor" of benefits but also toward containing costs by establishing new controls and promoting economy by encouraging new programs and incentives.

Fundamentally, however, the problems of Medicaid lie beyond the walls of Medicaid. The task force is strongly convinced that the current health system has serious organizational, financing, productivity, and access problems and that bolder moves than have characterized the last few years are needed to achieve measurable improvement. Appreciable investment of funds will be needed, but, importantly, significant changes in our delivery system are required. There are no easy solutions. The strategy of leadership and implementation will be complex inevitably, not only because the country is vast and diverse but also because the health field, like most human-service fields, lacks self-regulation and its traditions run deep. This suggests the desirability of building on the good that exists while seeking, selectively, levers for effecting change, utilizing the assets of the public and private sectors, neither of which, alone, can accomplish the job to be done.

The task force has no prescription for a new health-care

delivery system. The concept that any single formulation of resources could solve all the nation's health-care problems is as witless as the notion that a single remedy could cure all kinds of ailments. Thus, the task force has endorsed the Health Maintenance Organization (HMO) proposal[2] as an important step toward improvement in the organization and delivery of health services, not because it sees the HMO as the one best method of organizing services for the future or the one that should prevail but simply because it offers a promising option or alternative that may take its place in the system and vie with other methods on the basis of appropriateness of service and economy of performance.

This kind of competition among organizational modes within the system is regarded by the task force as desirable because it may stimulate performance by offering choices to both consumers and providers of care. But competition within the health-care system also has obvious risks. The first risk is that choices made by providers may be guided by self-interest and choices made by consumers may be misguided by ignorance. The second risk is that competition among organizational modes may of itself tend to separate the parts and obscure the view of the system as a whole; one man's pluralism is another man's incoherence.

To safeguard the system against the hazards of provider self-interest, consumer ignorance, and fragmentation, it must be managed. And the task force sees management of the system as given direction by Federal leadership—specifically in the Department of Health, Education, and Welfare. As it is envisioned and recommended here, the management function for the health-care system is to be innovative, but not prescriptive; bold, but not authoritarian. It is the intention that the federal leadership as far as possible shall guide, not direct; motivate, not demand; assist, not provide; and evaluate, not ordain.

With the necessary minimum of regulation, the manage-

---

[2] H.R. 17550, passed by the House of Representatives on May 21, 1970, and now pending in the Senate.

ment function is seen as formulating policy, establishing objectives, fashioning incentives, evaluating results, and, always, protecting and promoting the public interest—with the policies, goals, incentives, results, and public interest comprehending not just the Federal health programs and their beneficiaries, but the health-care system as a whole and the whole population.

Importantly, the task force believed that money spent for service must not accept uncritically the present mode of service nor by the pattern of spending sanctify it. Whether the source of funds is an individual, an insurance agency, or the Government, continual attempts must be made to reward effective service and penalize poor service through the design of payment, by incentives or by reference to such benchmarks as area-wide planning and accreditation.

Repeatedly it has been declared that the health system is in a crisis. More accurately it could be said instead that we have a system of crisis medicine created out of our failure to view health in broad social perspective. Health goals and services are keyed too often to institutional needs, not judged in terms of their impact on morbidity or mortality. If diet, inactivity, smoking, accidents, and pollution are significant causes of ill health, they must be brought within the sights of health agencies. Otherwise, the trade-offs required in the judicious use of scarce resources cannot be made rationally.

Hard as the task may be, the system must be oriented toward encouraging people to stay well, toward health maintenance, instead of only toward getting well. If the perspective of the health field is not broadened and if the orientation is not changed, we must be prepared to pay a larger price with a proportionately diminishing yield. The health field not only needs a strong infusion of money and effectiveness, it also needs a sounder philosophic framework and reevaluation of goals. The need for goals and programs to be formulated in a context broader than the dimensions of the health system itself was one of the major factors that convinced the task force that a separate Department of Health would not be wise at this time.

Other themes are identified in the body of the report, but one of these should be mentioned here. When one talks of the need for policy, goals, boundaries, trade-offs, and controls, the question arises as to who makes the ultimate decisions. The answer varies with the problem and, obviously, with the distinction between clinical and public policy situations. However, with more sophistication, greater access to the facts, and more experience, the consumer in health, as in education, wants a greater voice in matters affecting his well-being and his pocketbook. With the advent of massive public financing of health services through Congressional enactments in recent years, public decision making in the health services became inevitable, and public decision making without consumer participation is like an election without votes.

The task force believes that the day is past when doctors and hospital administrators and trustees and their associates may rely only on their own judgments of how they can best distribute all the skills and resources at their disposal to what they see as the greatest advantage for the people they think they should be serving. The resources today, in substantial part, are public or community resources, not excluding physicians trained largely at public expense; and their allocation and conditions of use are thus a public concern. The escalation from individual need to community crisis to public funding to public decision making is the choreography of social action in a democratic society. The task force is aware that some of the positions and maneuvers called for in the ballet impinge now on the traditions of a profession that prides itself on selectivity, rigorous training, and independent will; and the task force is concerned that leadership of the health services, federal and local, shall be prepared to accommodate the consumer interest with minimum abrasion.

Whether the result of consumer participation is a more relevant and responsive service, as the task force believes it can be, or unmitigated disaster, as many in the health professions believe will be the case, depends largely on leadership—the leadership of the individual institutions and programs and ultimately state and Federal programs, which must provide guidance and initiatives aimed at making consumer participation informed and responsible. It will not be easy. Many consumers are unaccustomed to working in an institutional framework. Progress can be slowed by conflicts within consumer ranks. Given reasonable and sympathetic support and direction, however, potentially more progress can be achieved with consumers expressing preference and need and at times resisting the eroding process of institutionalization.

These observations are intended to provide a background against which the recommendations can be seen more clearly. Because the task force represented a cross section of society in geography, age, profession, and consumer interest, the recommendations can be viewed as reflecting, albeit imperfectly, the mood of the country as a whole. Like the calls of crisis, they indicate clearly the need for affirmative and accountable public and managerial action ushering in a new era in the financing and delivery of health services—nothing less.

SUMMARY

The Big Ideas

The bedrock belief of the Task Force on Medicaid and Related Programs is that the American people should get more and better health care, and the means for providing it are at hand or can be developed.

It's a lot more complicated than that, obviously, but after a year of intensive study the task force recommendations, like a broad river whose flow is unaltered by cross currents and riptides, are all moving toward the one goal. For all their variety of subject and substance, the recommendations without exception relate in one way or another to the needs of consumers of health care, or the behavior of providers of health care, or the instruments, including money, that can identify the needs and guide the behavior. Thus, in fact there are three constellations of recommendations here, three big ideas, at times intertwined and at times divergent, but always on their way together toward achievement of the basic purpose.

Among the more than 125 specific recommendations in this report having to do with coverage and benefits, effectiveness, planning, management, financing, and such problems as long-term care and consumer participation in health affairs, the few that are summarized here can be identified more directly than the others with one or another of the big ideas. They're thus set apart in this synopsis, not because of a belief that by themselves they could accomplish the most toward achieving what the task force sees as the desirable objectives for the health service, but because they seem to furnish a navigation chart to task force thoughts.

Here is where we think the American health-care system should go, and here are the ways it can get there.

The first big idea is that all consumers should have access to health care without hardship or humiliation and, as far as possible, with some voice in how it is planned and some choice of how it is furnished.

The fact is that millions of consumers get care on a hit-or-miss basis; millions more lack access to care except in medical crises; and virtually all consumers lack access to the decision-making machinery that can bring about change. These gaps represent a failure of both public policy and private initiative. They are reflected in both public and private programs. The remedy cannot be found within the present structure of state Medicaid or without sweeping improvements in coverage and financing of private prepayment and insurance plans. The size of the gap in consumer access to the decision-making machinery of health care is apparent from the fact that few institutions and programs include users of their services on policy-making or governing boards, in spite of their nonprofit and, presumably, "community" character. The result is that medical care is still too often delivered at the time and place and in the way convenient to provider rather than consumer.

APPENDIX ONE

Old patterns persist in the face of new demands—a basic cause of rising dissatisfaction with the health services.

The following are a selection of our main recommendations related to the first big idea. The goals envisioned in them are seen as the least that can be done to redeem the promise of Medicaid that the poor and the near poor would be brought into the mainstream of American medicine and to give meaning to the declaration that access to medical care is a right of all.

We recommend converting Medicaid to a program with a uniform minimum level of health benefits financed one hundred percent by Federal funds, with a further Federal matching with states for certain types of supplementary benefits and for individuals not covered under the minimum plan.

First priority for protection under a basic Federal floor for Medicaid should be all persons eligible for payments under the proposed Family Assistance Plan. Additional groups should be phased in until all persons with incomes at or below the poverty level are covered.

Totally and permanently disabled Social Security beneficiaries should be included as soon as possible under title XVIII, Medicare.

Improvements in protection and administration of existing state Medicaid programs should not be delayed because of these possible later, larger Federal changes. Numerous opportunities for such improvements have been pinpointed.

Throughout its deliberations, the task force was deeply concerned that the very special needs of the aged for long-term institutional care are not being adequately provided in Medicaid or Medicare, even though the cost of the care that is provided has soared beyond expectations. Difficult problems of coverage and quality of care occur in the nursing home setting at the point where the need for medical services or supervision shades into the need for sensitive, personal, long-term care—a point that is difficult to define precisely and to determine even in the case of individual patients. The result has been that many patients needing continued care cannot get it because the needed care is personal or social, not medical; at the same time, institutions have been deprived of revenues when such determinations have been made retroactively. To resolve this complex of problems, the task force has recommended clearer separation of the medical and personal or social components of long-term care and re-examination of the methods of financing long-term care in relation to the financing of medical-care programs.

The Task Force recommends that the Department of Health, Education, and Welfare undertake further coordinated studies to develop policy which addresses directly the need for long-term care services and recognizes that a long-term care program has three components: (a) residential services; (b) personal support services; and (c) medical, dental, and psychiatric services.

The extended-care benefit in title XVIII (which is not a long-term care benefit) should be redefined and restructured to eliminate existing confusion and reduce administrative complexity.

The Department of Health, Education, and Welfare should give high priority to experiments involving referral and placement services, including the development of Community Placement Consultation Centers—a new concept to provide professional consultation regarding long-term care services and placement to all agencies and individuals in the community.

The task force is aware that this is the era of the consumer and that consumer organizations and representatives are making their influence felt in many ways in many aspects of society. Just as the universities are learning to live with the fact that their consumers are going to have a greater voice in shaping university programs, so must health institutions and programs learn to live with the fact that their consumers are going to have a real voice in planning and evaluating health services. While we recognize the inevitability of consumer participation and have seen examples of the valid contributions consumers have made to the effectiveness of health services, we are also aware of the misgivings of many health professionals who doubt that consumers can make substantive contributions and some who fear actual obstruction. The task force made these recommendations:

Any board or group set up to advise policy-making officials at any level of Government or of health-care agencies sponsored by Government must include consumer representatives to protect and present the interests and needs of the consumer. The consumer representatives selected to serve on policy-making and advisory boards should reflect the social, economic, racial, and geographic characteristics of their community.

Federal, state and non-governmental agencies involved in planning, delivering, and purchasing health services should make provision for special orientation programs for new members of policy-making groups, including the consumer representatives on such groups.

Programs of health education should be considered integral components of health-care services, and all providers receiving Federal support should be required to provide continuing programs of health education to their consumers.

The second big idea is that the health-care delivery system cannot function effectively in response to consumer demand and

provider self-interest but must be planned and managed so that the terms and conditions of payment shall have a powerful impact on the way the services are organized and delivered.

It is a central conclusion of the task force that money is needed but that money alone will not guarantee either capacity or effectiveness to the system. In fact, if a benevolent and affluent government were to begin to pay for all the basic health care needed by all those who can't pay for it themselves but no other change were introduced into the existing system, the result would be a disastrous rise in the cost of services that are already scarce. There isn't enough money and there aren't enough doctors to provide the needed care just on a fee-for-service basis; thus, any solution will require new options, new goals, and new attitudes. Without these, the health system cannot move forward to meet its growing responsibilities; with them, the task force is convinced that the recommendations in this report, most of which relate in one way or another to this big idea, can show the way toward achieving more and better health care for all Americans.

For two decades programs financing medical care, whether public or private, have been reinforcing traditional ways of providing service. The task force is convinced that it no longer makes sense to keep pouring new wine in old casks—some of which are leaking. Additional financing must be accompanied now, with opportunities and encouragement to physicians, hospitals, and others, to provide service in ways that permit a logical response to sound economic and patient-care incentives and to engage in a competition of organization and method.

The task force believes that the methods of reimbursement and conditions of participation in Medicare and Medicaid and the investment policies of all Federal financing programs are the best instruments for achieving increased capacity and new organizational patterns in the delivery of health services. Moreover, "front-end" or "start-up" money at this early stage is crucial.

APPENDIX ONE

The Federal Government should provide leadership and funds to create and support systems of health care, through a variety of auspices and approaches, that will contain the following desirable elements: (1) comprehensive services and continuity of care; (2) defined population groups which contract for services; (3) integrated fiscal and managerial responsibility; and (4) sharing risk through prepayment.

Legislation should be enacted to make sums equivalent to five percent of Federal Medicaid appropriations each year available for the development and improvement of health-care services and resources. Priorities should be given to development of organized primary health-care services, especially in neighborhoods with a high proportion of low-income persons; to development of services and resources which can serve as alternatives to inpatient hospital care, e.g., home-health-care programs; to improvements in utilization, efficiency, and quality of existing facilities and services; to social and other outreach services integral to appropriate utilization of medical services; and to development of ways to link and relate new and existing health services with each other aiming toward comprehensive health-care systems in communities.

The task force strongly endorses the innovative approach of the Administration's Health Maintenance Organization proposal to provide an option for Medicare and Medicaid beneficiaries to elect to receive health services through a single organization that provides coordinated services financed through prepaid capitation.

Reimbursements to hospitals and other providers of service under Medicare and Medicaid should be on a prospective instead of a retrospective basis, thereby offering providers the motivation to retain savings that come from economies effected as well as to bear the risk of costs incurred beyond agreed rates.

There should be active support for the principles of the legislative amendments on incentive reimbursement and the other provisions in the Administration's Health Cost Effectiveness proposals. HEW should actively program experiments for incentive reimbursement under Medicare and Medicaid with new emphasis on experiments in payment methods for physicians, the key generators of health service utilization.

The third big idea is that the whole has to be more than the sum of the parts. The health service system must be more than the aggregate of all the personal transactions among consumers and providers. If capacities are to be increased in keeping with demand and effectiveness improved in keeping with responsible practice, the system must have a guiding intelligence—not laid on from outisde but designed and ingrained into the way the system operates.

We keep hearing anguished cries about the "fragmentation" of health service as though this were some new and monstrous thing, but the fact is that fragmentation began when the doctor could no longer get everything he needed in his saddle-bags and has been going on ever since, an inevitable result of the increasingly specialized technology. Fragmentation of services may be unavoidable at times and, of itself, is not always bad. What is bad is that for lack of overall leadership we have allowed organization and management to become fragmented, along with service, to the point where patients may be handed off from one institution or service or program to another in a kind of medical bucket line, with nobody in charge determining where the line begins, which way it goes, and where it ends. The result is that cost mounts and care suffers, not just for the poor but for the whole population. To find the beginning, chart the way, and determine the end will require leadership not just of the parts but of the whole.

The task force believes this leadership is the proper role of the Federal Government.

To achieve effective planning in capital investment and manpower development, to use purchasing power to stimulate and support innovations in the health delivery system, and to avoid duplication and counter-productive use of resources, the health component of the Department of Health, Education, and Welfare should be further strengthened to provide a full capability for goals setting, planning, and coordination of major health policies. This includes establishing an under secretary for health and scientific affairs and a health systems analysis planning staff in his office to serve as the motive force for analysis and planning and as the permanent staff for a council of health advisors (recommended).

There is an urgent need to establish a National Council of Health Advisors responsible for assessing the nation's health status and the status of the health system, for assisting in generating national health goals, and for outlining health-care objectives applicable generally to Federal health programs. The council would consist of a small number of people broadly representative and highly qualified, having a public point of view, and appointed by the President. The council should report to the secretary of HEW and issue an annual report to the nation.

Good progress has been made recently in the revitalization, reorganization, and staffing of the Medical Services Administration, the agency administering the Medicaid program at the Federal level, but substantial additional administrative resources must be provided for this program at central, regional, and state levels.

The department should develop model systems and procedures for the states, and they should be required to adopt medicaid program-effectiveness systems designed to control over- and under-utilization; assure that payment and eligibility determinations are appropriate; encourage efficient planning, evaluation, and administration; and aid in determining that sufficient resources are available and accessible to provide adequate services to recipients and provide data to meet Federal requirements.

Planning is the key to achieving high-quality services that maximize consumer satisfaction and, as well, safeguard professional concerns and the general public interest to make the most effective use of scarce dollars.

The Federal Government, through the Department of Health, Education, and Welfare, should clarify the goals, function, and authority of local Comprehensive Health Service Planning Agencies and assure adequate funding to create effective agencies covering all important areas.

Local comprehensive planning agencies should not be saddled with broad decision-making powers. Instead, the local agencies should be viewed as playing an advisory, consultative, facilitative role. Final authority to franchise health facilities, allocate investment resources, and approve project grants should not rest with the local or state planning agency but rather with the governor or some other publicly accountable entity—or in the case of decisions bearing on the amount of third-party or Federal reimbursement, with the third party or with HEW, as the case may be.

Consonant with the conviction that it is the whole system, and not just parts of it, that must eventually be seen in total perspective, the task force considered that there may be many additional millions in the population not eligible for benefits under any of the existing or recommended program extensions but who are also subject at times to heavy medical expense exceeding the limits of family resources and of protection

APPENDIX ONE

afforded by available prepayment or insurance coverage. Recommendations as to the desirability of a national health insurance plan or the merits of any of the specific plans that have been proposed would have carried us beyond the scope of responsibility of this task force. Nevertheless, our discussions and recommendations had to comprehend the relationship between possible future financing programs and the health-care delivery system.

We recommend that the Secretary appoint a high-level body to undertake promptly a study directed toward the development of a health-care financing policy for the nation.

Included in our report are: (1) a list of central and necessary objectives against which we believe long-range financing proposals should be measured; and (2) a set of specific issues and questions by which different proposals can be compared and appraised.

APPENDIX TWO

In response to the CBS documentaries on health care in America, the American Medical Association took immediate action to present its side. The following are reprints of the *AMA Newsletter* and a story that appeared in the *Medical World News*.

Special Issue, April 22, 1970

AMA took immediate action to secure equal television time in order to rebut the distorted picture of American medicine as presented Monday and Tuesday by the CBS network in two programs called "The Promise and the Practice" and "Don't Get Sick in America."

AMA's board of trustees, meeting April 24, will give special attention to the association's long-term communications needs and finances following the CBS attack on medicine.

The programs gave millions of viewers the impression that the nation's physicians are unwilling to attempt to solve health care problems, and that the solution must therefore be turned over to the government.

Telegrams were sent to William S. Paley, chairman of the CBS board, and to Richard Salant, CBS president, following each of the telecasts. Monday night's wire read: "We request equal time to present one hour documentary on health care in USA portraying positive efforts being made to improve health care which your documentary . . . carefully avoided . . ." It was signed by AMA President Gerald D. Dorman, M.D., and NMA President Julius W. Hill, M.D. The two issued a second appeal following Tuesday night's telecast. The second telegram read: "Your CBS health care program . . . was far less a documentary than an editorial in support of compulsory government medicine. We repeat our request for equal time to present a balanced story. It is our conviction that our request should be approved in the public interest and in the interest of fair play."

Copies of the wires were sent to Dean Burch, chairman of the Federal Communications Commission, with a letter from AMA's EVP stating the association's case for equal time. CBS had not replied as of noon Wednesday. In Tuesday's New York *Daily News*, Salant was quoted as saying the network considers the programs to be "fair, accurate, and an important public service."

Press releases were issued by AMA following each program. Chicago *Daily News* noted AMA's request for equal time to present "the many positive efforts being made to improve American health care." The *News* commented that the AMA's proposed program sounds "exceptionally interesting."

In a joint statement after Monday night's program, both medical association presidents declared the programs "underscored only the negative, thereby stimulating angry feelings of frustration—and offered no solutions except a nebulous health care plan."

The slant of the programs was clearly indicated by the producer, Burton Benjamin, just before the shows were broadcast. He said the shows do not endorse alternatives, adding: "But the alternatives are obvious. Group health plans are increasing in popularity in this country, and beyond that, some sort of national health plan is needed."

In a statement issued Wednesday, Dr. Dorman and Dr. Hill declared that the second presentation of the series was "slanted, totally unbalanced and a disservice to medicine." They also said: "We now believe the American public is entitled to a fair, balanced presentation of a social issue of this magnitude. Certainly the public has a right to know the whole truth."

AMA was not permitted to preview the shows. However, warnings that the programs were scheduled and probably would be highly critical of medicine were carried in the *AMA Newsletter* on March 2 and March 30, in Operations Grassroots resource material on April 8, and in *American Medical News*. A telegram was sent April 16 to alert all medical societies. AMA is preparing television spots that will be mailed next week to state and county medical societies with CBS affiliates. Dr. Dorman and Dr. Hill will each be featured in one-minute spots, and a five-minute spot will bring messages from both presidents.

Local medical societies are urged to protest immediately to their CBS affiliate stations, showing the AMA telegrams to Paley and Salant to the station managers. Each society in an area with a CBS affiliate station should consider requesting time to respond to the programs. Advertising copy is being prepared by the AMA and will be sent this week to state and local medical societies. The ads are suggested

The CBS Television Mess—Morris Fishbein, M.D.

With many preliminary announcements and great furor, the Columbia Broadcasting System recently ushered in a two-evening program called "Health in America."

After the first evening's program the TV critic of the *New York Times*, Jack Gould, predicted that the medical profession would howl loudly about what he asserted was a presentation of facts. One indication that his prediction had some validity was an announcement by the AMA and the National Medical Association that they wanted equal time to respond.

I wasted two hours of *my* prime time watching these programs. It is very probable that I know more of the facts than does the critic of the *Times*, and I must assert that the programs were not factual. By grouping certain items together it gave false impressions of the actual situation. For example, a view of the AMA building was accompanied by adjectives indicating that it is a palatial edifice, and that just a short distance away are slums where people live without medical care. In all fairness, this could be said with equal truth about the White House in our nation's capital. In his review of the TV program, Gould called it a "biting" two-evening series, and he referred to the "lush" headquarters of the AMA—examples of how words can carry bias.

The primary theme of the first hour was continuous condemnation of the medical profession. It was criticized because it was said to be mercenary, because doctors move to the suburbs rather than residing in the slums, because they do not make house calls, because their bills are high—indeed a mustering of all the points of attack used by those who are demanding reform. The second hour criticized insurance and told of the advantages of group practice.

Anyone experienced in modern journalism in the U.S. knows how a story or news report can be slanted. By accumulating reports of dramatic incidents and publishing them all at one time, the public can be alarmed and be made to think in terms of an epidemic of such incidents.

Better Balance Needed

A balanced account of health in America might have included at least a glimpse of the NIH and its widespread activities. A view of Massachusetts General Hospital and even the almost-moribund Cook County Hospital could have shown, in addition to overcrowded outpatient facilities, the swift attention given under different circumstances to emergency situations. Perhaps a little balance might have been secured by some photographs from England with its national health system, or from Russia with its state-controlled medicine, indicating some of the obvious difficulties under which both these nations operate in delivering high-quality medical care.

However, CBS did not want a balanced presentation. Apparently the producer wanted to arouse the public against not only the AMA but the whole profession. Unmentioned was the fact that while labor strives for a thirty-five-hour week, many a doctor works fifty to sixty hours a week or more.

While there are slum areas with only one or two doctors to care for many thousands of people, at close hand are the medical services of such great hospitals as Johns Hopkins, New York Hospital, Massachusetts General, Billings Hospital, Michael Reese Hospital, and literally a thousand others. The people who use these outpatient services know about them. Unfortunately, some either are unaware of their availability or, through apathy, never reach them. But the inclusion of this kind of information in the CBS presentation would have defeated the sensational approach.

Many people are predicting that American TV, as now practiced, is in a decline and perhaps approaching an even greater reorganization and control than confronts the medical profession. Even in the face of this, though, which of the networks will take two hours to show the difficulties of American TV? To reveal its emphasis on soap operas or the way in which discussion programs are used as sounding boards for ambitious politicos? To demonstrate the difficulty of securing equal time when an individual or an entire industry or profession is submitted to a biased exhibition of its frailties?

Granted, honest, factual presentation of any situation is difficult; that is inherent in the system. But the system can be changed, just as the medical profession, hospitals, health insurance agencies, and methods of medical practice are constantly undergoing change. Perhaps that was the major difficulty with the production of "Health in America." It seems to have been a hastily concocted, scrappy, disconnected, incomplete, and wholly unsatisfactory display of either health or medicine in America. In a word, it was a mess.

APPENDIX THREE

The two CBS Reports' documentaries caused a major controversy. Many people wrote congratulating CBS for enlightening the public to the "sorry" state of the American healthcare system; many were indignant because they believed CBS was degrading the time-honored medical profession; and many were upset because they felt CBS was advocating socialized medicine. Here is a sampling of the many letters CBS received:

22 April 1970

MR. DANIEL SHORE
CBS
CHICAGO, ILL.

Sir,
I am a Chicago graduate and was in general practice (M.D.) in Mt. Prospect, Illinois, from 1927 till my semi-retirement in 1965. I now live in Iron Ridge and Hustisford, Wis. This area is well supplied with doctors and hospitals; I am not too busy nor want to be, for reasons of health.

I saw your 20th. and 21st. April, 9 P.M. program. I congratulate you and the CBS on this program and hope it will get some desired results. Publicity and more publicity is needed to awaken the government and the A.M.A. who can remedy the disgraceful situation so many citizens of the richest nation in the world are in. We have too many chiefs and too few warriors. The shortage of family doctors is the most important and immediate problem. A humble general practitioner dares to give the influential A.M.A. a simple solution which would immediately begin to show results and within four years give all the people in every locality, urban and rural, easy access to medical help.

1-Lower entrance requirements to pre-medical schools.

2-Decrease the pre-medical course from four to one year; in my time it was two years.

3-Decrease the medical course from four to three years. Many subjects are given in too much detail for an education in general medicine.

4-Only a six months general internship.

5-Finally and most important, require a one year general practice period in a government dictated location before issuing a final license.

A total saving of at least three and one half years. Practical experience is more important than book knowledge which can be acquired at the same time. This graduate would be well-qualified to treat 90% of all office and home patients.

The government subsidizes every medical student who pays only a small amount of the actual cost of his education, so the government has a right to enforce this one year requirement and military service.

All post graduate work, needed and desired, for specialization may then follow. Teaching experience, during this time, would be invaluable to the student and the school. Years ago an intern received no salary, now he gets from $500 to $1000 per month. That is why most students become specialists; no incentive to get out and work.

What did the medical profession do to make general practice more appealing to the students? It increased the medical education by two or three years so we would have "specialists" in family practice. Sensible?

The A.M.A. will continue on its usual course; the government must initiate action, and now. You and the news media can get results.

Wish you luck.

Sincerely yours,
Alfred Wolfarth, M.D.

P.S.
I would be happy to answer any questions. You may quote me any way you wish.

April 22, 1970

Gentlemen:

I did catch the second in the three part series "Health in America" which dealth with the spiraling costs of Medical Treatment.

It was indeed worthwhile viewing. I was thoroughly impressed with the program in general.

Since, I am involved in Health Care, the program was of special interest to me.

Unquestionably, something must be done and soon to alleviate this high cost for medical care.

APPENDIX THREE

I thoroughly disagree with the President of The Medical Association, who stated that yes, something should be done but not for five or ten years. He stated that we were not ready. Who is not ready? The doctors perhaps. The sick people and their families are ready right now.

I particularly, enjoyed and readily concurred with Professor Rashi Fein. He struck me as a very remarkable man with the proper insight into this most serious, pressing problem.

I hope he, and others like him, can be instrumental in bringing to the people of this Country improved Health Services. Improved in not only cost but quality.

The quality of Health Service today leaves much to be desired.

Sincerely,
(Mrs.) J.B. Sussina, R.N. B.S.

April 22, 1970

MR. DANIEL SHORE
CBS REPORTS
COLUMBIA BROADCASTING SYSTEM
51 W. 52ND STREET
NEW YORK, N.Y. 10019

RE: "Don't Get Sick In America"

Dear Mr. Shore:

I watched your news special on "Don't Get Sick In America" stated what our problems are in our present health care system. Certainly the hospital plays a major role in our health care delivery and will perhaps play an increasing role in the future.

However, I feel that there were several things which were not pointed out in the program and perhaps could be covered in a future program.

First of all, I think it should be pointed out that our Medicare and Medicaid Programs are based on hospital cost in providing services. Anytime you base a program on cost, there are no incentives for the hospital running or trying to run an efficient organization. In fact, the penalties for an efficient organization are the decreases in the percentage of reimbursements per patient. The American Hospital Association has been working with the Social Security Administration for several years in recognizing some of the problems in their reimbursement system.

I also felt you neglected to state what the private voluntary sector is doing about these problems pointed out in your program. You did mention the Kaiser Foundation Program, but you did not cite what some of the community hospitals are doing about their problems in delivering health care.

I happen to be in one of these community hospitals in the private voluntary sector of health care. Our community has been well aware of its problems in the delivery of health care for at least the past 5 years. One of these is that we have two general acute, non-profit hospitals operating within the city—St. Mary's Hospital, 227 beds and Wausau Memorial Hospital, 140 beds. I am enclosing a news clipping from our local newspaper covering the story of the hospital merger where both hospital boards of directors have recently agreed to merge into one hospital corporation.

I know that the hospital merger in Wausau, Wisconsin, is being duplicated in many communities throughout the United States. The only goal in merging facilities is to provide the best possible care to the citizens of the area at the least possible cost. I am sure you can recognize the competition between hospitals in one community, or communities relatively close to each other, is not desirable in meeting the present day needs of our delivery of health care. The most striking needs in the nation's hospitals today is *health manpower*. Our merger in Wausau will consolidate the health manpower of the two hospitals and thereby provide better and more efficient utilization of health manpower to the patients served by the new corporation. The hospital merger will eliminate duplication of services and facilities.

The sharing of services was touched on by Mr. Berke, President of the American Hospital Association, on your program last night, but the merging of hospitals was not covered at all. I think this area of the health care field certainly deserves mention.

Sincerely,
Stewart W. Laird

APPENDIX THREE

April 22, 1970

CBS NEWS SERVICE
CBS TELEVISION
NEW YORK, NEW YORK

Dear Sirs:

Your efforts in behalf of the socialization of medicine were truly remarkable. It is hoped that your next effort will be on the socialization or nationalization of the communications media, particularly television.

Sincerely yours,
G. S. Barnes, M.D.

April 22, 1970

RICHARD S. SALANT
PRESIDENT, C.B.S. NEWS
C.B.S. BUILDING
AVENUE OF THE AMERICAS
NEW YORK, NEW YORK

Dear Sir:

I saw the Don't Get Sick in America program and I was terribly disappointed in it. It was strongly biased as I'm sure you meant it to be but it was so unfair.

You blamed most of the ills of medical care on the ancient system of delivery. You failed to mention what most people overlook that the vast majority of sick people are taken care of not in hospitals but in doctors' offices. Hospital administrators like for the public to believe otherwise.

You stated that many doctors received over twenty-five thousand dollars a year and a few over one hundred thousand a year. You failed to mention that the A.M.A. has tried unsuccessfully to get the government to release the names of the doctors who collect these large sums. You failed to mention that in one case, at least, the doctor returned over one hundred thousand dollars and when his practice was investigated it was found that his charges were earned and the state returned the money to him. You failed to mention that every state has utilization committees working to ferret out the misuse of these funds. You failed to mention that before medicaid was started in any state actuaries of insurance companies testified as did the A.M.A. that the money appropriated for medicaid couldn't possibly cover the cost.

The brilliant people on your staff surely know that the level of education determines the standard of medical care. When someone said that our medical care is inadequate he failed to mention that some of the highest infant mortality rates in these states are within a stones throw of Johns Hopkins Hospital in Baltimore, St. Lukes in New York, Michael Reese in Chicago. The lack of proper medical care is due more to ignorance, indifference and apathy than to lack of facilities or indifference on the part of physicians.

When you showed the picture of Kaiser-Permanente growing at the rate of ten percent a year you failed to mention that many areas and hospitals are growing as much or more. Certainly we need more motel-like facilities where people may go for tests—many hospitals already have them—but you failed to mention that. It's unfortunate that you used Kaiser-Permanente as a model because its many deficiencies almost but not quite negate its good points.

In your scorn of the A.M.A. I believe you were unfair and you certainly do a disservice to the medical profession. Incidentally, you along with other organizations that are so critical and sometimes even vitriolic against the A.M.A. and physicians in general are doing the only thing you can to discourage young people going into medicine. If I didn't know any more about the A.M.A. than you indicated on your program Tuesday night I'd be ashamed to practice medicine.

Many changes are occurring in the delivery of medical care. One county in Virginia couldn't persuade patients to get in buses to come to the county seat so clinics were opened in population centers over the county. Now one day a week—a pediatrician, an orthopedist, a dentist, a nutritionist, and a social service worker not to mention residents and interns conduct a clinic in these out of the way places. Each day over one hundred children are examined and treated. This is a departure that our small county hopes to emulate.

You Don't Get Sick in America I think is a disgraceful affair and certainly beneath the level of coverage I'd expect from one of the three major networks. It upsets me because I am an honest, hard-working, earnest doctor as the vast majority of physicians are and I think you pictured us as arrogant, money-grabbing, entrepreneurs (that was the word one of your speakers used.) I resent the idea.

Very truly yours,
George D. Johnson, M.D.

APPENDIX THREE

April 22, 1970

EDITOR
CBS NEWS
NEW YORK, N.Y.

Dear Sir:
Your two-part program "Don't Get Sick in America" was certainly attention-getting and interesting. In the interest of good reporting with some editorializing, I would suggest several points that could have been emphasized a bit:

Item I—The immigrant with the kidney failure retained his foreign citizenship—and remigrated. Of necessity, any one who cannot pay for his own medical care has that care omitted or subsidized by others. In fairness, should American taxpayers subsidize a foreigner? Any foreigner? To what number of dollars! Do the European countries subsidize American citizens resident there in a comparable manner?

Item II—Wolcott, Indiana has a problem—as do hundreds of comparable small communities in the USA. The problem is indeed regrettable. Need I point out for emphasis that any law of the USA that could require a physician to practice in an area not of his own choosing could also require the residents of such a community to live elsewhere—where physicians were available. I believe that such law would conflict with the involuntary servitude to our constitution, as well as depriving the physician of his freedom to be a citizen of the USA, and his right to live and work where he chooses.

Item III—Re: The Wolcott, Indiana family that was unable to get a night time house call for their sick child—diagnosis appendicitis. I don't know of any physician who carries the tools for an appendectomy in his black bag. A house call in such cases may be reassuring to the parents, but would result in further delay in obtaining necessary surgical care. A group practice set-up as you seem to favor could not have put the doctor closer to Wolcott than the geography would permit. In fact, considering the sparse population, the distance for a group practice might even be increased in a case such as this.

Item IV—The lack of physicians living and practicing in the so-called ghetto areas is most distressing, and does work hardships on many of the ghetto residents. Do any CBS newsmen live in these areas? Do they enter these areas at night alone?

DON'T GET SICK IN AMERICA

Willingly? As a matter of choice? Most American citizens would be terrified at the thought of living or working in such areas—especially those citizens such as physicians who are attractive targets for hold-up and robberies, since they are assumed to possess money in their pockets and narcotics in their black bags. Did it ever occur to the CBS News staff that placing doctors in the ghetto areas at night might reduce the already short supply of doctors? It is not the physician, who are concerned Americans, who make the inner core of the cities such undesirable places to live in or work in. I believe it is the residents of such areas who make the areas what they are. Certainly there is no easy answer to that problem.

Item V—There has been and still are dedicated physicians who work in these areas. The major part of their income is from welfare, medicare, or medicaid funds. Now, certain of our senators have seen fit to single out physicians who have billed or collected $25,000 or more in a single year from these public assistance programs, and have implied that these doctors are suspected of being criminals and crooks. Such attitude on the part of U.S. Senators is unlikely to inspire physicians "to take up the torch," and carry it there where he is so much needed; and then be publically villified for so doing. Do you believe that these senators are trying to help the unfortunate ghetto residents?

Do you think it was fair to title a two-hour news program aimed at all of USA on the case of a single foreigner suffering from a very unusual and uncommon disease? Was this case typical? I believe that if CBS had tried they could have found many examples of good and fairly-priced medical services; perhaps even a majority of Americans might be well satisfied—at least it would make an interesting study for CBS to undertake.

If you wish to quote or comment publicly on this letter you have my permission; also permission to use my name. In fairness to me, I would request that quotes, if made, be kept in context.

Sincerely,
Lucian A. Arata, M.D.

April 20, 1970

Dear Sirs,
It is 10:00 p.m. Our children are in bed asleep and for the past hour I have watched -alone - your documentary on American

APPENDIX THREE

Medicine. I watched this program tonight and countless other programs on countless other nights sitting alone - because my husband is a physician - a General Practitioner in a rural community. He left the house early this morning - returned home for dinner at 7:30 and by 8:00 p.m. was gone again. He'll sleep at the hospital tonight (if circumstances permit sleep) and then he will try to get home before the children leave for school tomorrow. Then off to the office for another day.

I will be the first to admit that there are many things wrong with medical care in America. But why, why must the practicing physician always bear the blame and the shame? It saddens those of us personally involved to always be blamed and to hear you advocate the only solution as a government controlled program of medicine.

This will certainly not attract more young men to choose a profession in medicine. Instead, it will drive potential doctors and practicing physicians away from the practice of medicine. Perhaps I should rejoice - the government might insist that my husband limit himself to a 40 hour week!

Medicare and Medicaide have already forced extra hours of paperwork on already overworked doctors. How do you think a doctor must feel after spending 24 years and thousands of dollars to educate himself - then to be told by a clerk in the medicare office what procedures he can or can not do. What drugs he may or may not prescribe. That he can not charge what he feels is a fair price for his services? This can not compensate for the fact that he is now getting paid for services he once gave free.

Doctors are all too often presented on programs such as yours as money-hungry, high-living parasites.

There are still doctors who selected their profession for the more noble reasons.

We were married and had 2 children when my husband started his medical education. This involved 7 years of hard work, long separations from his family and sacrifice. It meant both of us working, borrowing every penny possible and the loss of his regular income for 7 years.

My husband was 38 years old before he started to practice. While our contemparies had homes, furniture and fine automobiles - we had debts and more debts. But we had made an investment in our future and America's future. Those years spent in training can never be recovered, but we felt the investment was worth the long hours, money and heartaches we put into my husband's medical education. We did not have wealthy parents or a wealthy government to pay for his education. We're proud we did it ourselves - The American Way!

We hope to have his medical education paid for by the time our children start to college.

We would have never made the effort had we known that instead of being able to fulfill a dream of practicing medicine - and all of those old-fashion sentiments concerned - our only future now is one of government control of his practice. Being told eventually (as you seem to advocate) where to live, how to practice and just whom he must treat.

Believe me, this is *not* our dream!

This way of life holds no appeal for us. After all of our sacrifices and dreams - we would desert the practice of medicine rather than submit to the type of medicine you advocate.

Regardless of how trite it sounds, you can't mass-produce doctors. There must be a dedication, desire, determination *and* ability. No man prepares this long or works this hard for the promise of a good income. Money can't buy the dedication and devotion my husband feels for his work and his patients.

I cry tonight for an American dream lost - For countless thousands who view the M.D. thru the eyes of C.B.S. News.

Sorrowfully,
Mrs. Carl T. Duer

April 21, 1970

Gentlemen:
 I do not believe that I have ever seen a *more biased or one sided* view of health care and the health profession in all of

APPENDIX THREE

my life as I witnessed on your TV show "Health Care in America" April 20, 1970.

Believe me this country needs help fast when a major TV network can tell so many half-truths and twisted, distorted staged interviews and get away with it without being charged under the "truth in packaging" laws. The bottom of the barrel has been scraped by you so long as you now have a hole in it.

C. Graham

April 24, 1970

CBS TV
NEW YORK CITY, NEW YORK

Gentlemen:

Thank you for your program "Don't Get Sick in America". It's been long past due. Having had a great deal of chronic illness in our family of five, we have had much first hand experience with doctors. Two of them have been really dedicated and wonderful human beings who have not tried to take advantage of our illnesses. The others—at least eight I can remember—have been interested only in their inflated fees being collected at the least possible inconvenience to them. I am a very conservative Republican, but would vote for socialized medicine today if given the opportunity.

Yours very truly,
Mrs. Paul M. Peterson

April 21, 1970

COLUMBIA BROADCASTING SYSTEMS
NEW YORK, N.Y.

Attn: Mr. Daniel Schorr

Three cheers for CBS concerning the latest report concerning Health in America and the discerning interrogative reporting conducted in presenting the facts and opinions. There can be little doubt that such a service has been long overdue in a Nation which has apparently lost its sense of values.

Our overall programs concerning Viet-Nam, Foreign Aid, Space Program must be curtailed in order to meet the pressing problems of ecology, health, and housing improvement. The pot of dissension continues to boil in the minds of the masses and the results could be most horrendous unless Government perceives the urgency to do something concrete before it is too late.

I am convinced that the viewers of the program could differentiate the degree of integrity and the false statements of those interviewed. The politicians will have to accept the fact that America is growing up and the intelligence quotient is increasing in geometric progression and giving the layman a grasp of events and facts which can not be so easily distorted by spokesmen of pressure groups. People are beginning to look at themselves and wonder how defeated nations such as Germany and Japan along with other Western Nations are enjoying economic stability with Health Programs and full employment while we blindly attempt to convert the world to some superficial image.

Americans have the right to good Health and are grateful of your efforts in bringing this matter more forcibly to the attention of our leaders.

Sincerely,
Carl W. Olson

April 20, 1970

PRESIDENT RICHARD M. NIXON
THE WHITE HOUSE
WASHINGTON 25, D.C.

Dear President Nixon:
I am writing in desperation to say, in effect, that it is strangling for one to find that he cannot accept life in his own time. My husband and I are hoping that you and Vice-President Agnew feel, as we do, that this evening's CBS program on medical care should have been labeled an editorial.
It has been for some time an overwhelming temptation for me to voice my feelings on health care in the state of Louisiana, my native state and my present place of residence. The charity hospital system in this state must surely rival, if not surpass, any in our country. Certainly, people must wait for attention; there are many who are ill. But, there are also many standing in these long lines who have just decided they had better get "checked" because they have a headache or because they have a garden variety cold. My puzzlement abounds when I find our state, reputedly quite adequate in its handling of health

APPENDIX THREE

care for the poor, swallowed up into federal programs, unbelievably full of red tape and misinformation, handled by people unfamiliar with our area. My source authority is my husband, who, at the age of 30, just began a pediatrics practice, having received all of his clinical training in our charity hospitals. My husband and I have both worked hard so that he might become a thoroughly trained pediatrician. He spent three years in undergraduate training, four years in medical schooling, one year in internship, two years in residency, and two years as a United States Air Force pediatrician. During his schooling and training, I taught school, leaving a baby at home. Is it wrong that he be compensated monetarily? The only difference between him and an electrician, as a measure of manpower, is that the electrician probably worked today from 8 a.m. until 5 p.m. My husband worked from 8 a.m. until 6 p.m., left home again at 9 p.m. It is 11 p.m. now, and I don't know yet when he will be home again. Is it wrong that I expect society to judge my husband as a kind and just person until he proves himself otherwise? I speak with authority as a doctor's daughter and a doctor's wife when I say that when charity care is indicated to these doctors in my life it is given generously. Never have I known my father or my husband to neglect a person in need. If many in their profession did, there could be many psychotic doctors who could not live with themselves.

Does it occur to the "powers that be" in Washington that:

1. A socialized medical system can only create 8 to 5'ers in the medical profession?
2. The threat of an impending socialization could be scaring prospective doctors away from medical schools?
3. It is not the threat of a lesser income that worries doctors generally; it is blind, massive government control over a profession that can seldom afford the time to involve itself in government and therefore would have no real vote?
4. The misled public expects "today's" medicine in the horse and buggy tradition (e.g. the plea for house calls, which is ridiculous because of necessary untransportable equipment and believe it or not, frequently physical danger for the physician)?

In summary, I am very much interested in your attitude toward our problem. When CBS chooses the more populous cities in the nation and treats their medical problems and ours in a lump, it appears unfair, biased, and misleading. We must have some recourse. What can you offer us?

DON'T GET SICK IN AMERICA

Thank you for your attention. I am, my dear Mr. President,

Sincerely yours,
Mrs. H.N. Winterton, Jr.
cc: CBS News
   c/o Columbia Broadcasting System
   51 W. 52nd. Street
   New York, New York 10019

April 22, 1970

DANIEL SHORE,
C/O CBS TELEVISION SERIES, "HEALTH IN AMERICA"
NEW YORK, N.Y.

Dear Mr. Shore:

I'd like to say that this is the most important series ever aired on television. It wasn't until the government became involved with this nation's health care that the people had a chance to be heard on the issue of medical care in America.

Of course, the American Medical Association don't want it. Does anybody want to cut down the money tree? Britain didn't want it either - I mean the BMA didn't want it but it has worked in Britain in spite of what the AMA says about it and in this poor nation even their system beats the hell out of ours. And I should know.

Why has the AMA never investigated the West German, the Dutch, the Scandinavian, or the Japanese systems and commented on them? Because they work so well and they don't want to know about it.

I had first hand knowledge of the British system. We were stationed at an Air Base near Oxford a number of years. An old case of tuberculosis of mine became re-activated. My English doctor said so long as my husband was doing his bit for the defense of the west, I was entitled to National Health care. He put me into a small private room at The Osler Sanatorium. I got the finest TB drugs to be had and the finest nursing and medical care, X-rays, drugs, room, nursing and everything was free to me. I got well. Not arrested. Well.

No National Health System is free to native citizens. They pay for it on a salary deduction basis but it is not missed. After all, we pay insurance premiums for health care, don't we? Social Security is a salary deducted, matched by government money. Why isn't it Socialized Security - like the big bad name, Socialized Medicine?

APPENDIX THREE

Our money pays for medical research but we cannot afford its benefits. Could a southern sharecropper afford intensive care in any hospital? How can poor people afford care in a hospital *room* which costs from $30,000 to $50,000 to build.

Let me ask you another question. If the medical profession is so overworked how come the AMA intends to support legal abortions? Because, again, this is a money tree. It is in Japan and it is in England. Do you think these doctors are going to pass up that good money?

Thanks for bringing this program to us.

Sincerely yours
Mrs. H. K. MacCorkle

April 23, 1970

MR. DANIEL SHORE
CBS TV NEWS
NEW YORK, NEW YORK

Dear Mr. Shore:

I cannot in good conscience allow your recent TV series on physicians and hospitals to go without comment.

While not a working newsman, I do have both a Bachelor's and a Master's degree in journalism and so am somewhat qualified to recognize the difference between thorough reporting and really cursory reporting.

I feel that your two TV specials fell in the latter category inasmuch as they were very thorough and very complete in covering the things that served your particular purpose. However, they were not objective, but one-sided and biased.

You neglected to point out that the medical care available in the United States is unquestionably the best available in the world. Certainly it has its faults, but there are many, many men and women working hard to change those areas that are in need of change. It's still the best system there is available, South Africa and its first heart transplant notwithstanding. They had to come to the United States to learn about a better way to repair damaged hearts.

It is very simple to find fault with an existing system. We found that out when Mr. Agnew attacked the TV and total news reporting system. It is much more difficult to propose adequate, viable solutions. I would have appreciated it had you been impartial enough to at least suggest that there were solutions, but that takes a little more time and a little more effort, doesn't it?

DON'T GET SICK IN AMERICA

How about a series now on what's good about American medicine? I am sure that you could fill two hours just as easily.

Sincerely,
Joseph W. Lindner

"DON'T GET SICK IN AMERICA"
CBS NEWS
51 W. 52ND
NEW YORK, NEW YORK

Dear Sir:
In my opinion your broadcast on the above subject was horrible beyond measure.

In the first place, California's prices are far beyond the national average. Locally, the daily room is a little less than half what you quoted.

Secondly, the doctors I know work far longer hours than anyone else is willing to do. I had a broken neck, with many years (15) of therapy and two operations. I can attest to their skill, kindness, and understanding during that entire time.

My brother in Ft. Worth has just completed a series of cobalt treatments for cancer. All the people in Ft. Worth go to this one center; and I know of a similar situation in many cities. You certainly did not give this side of the picture.

On what do you base your allegation that the U.S. has the poorest health of any western country? Whose statistics do you use? You were careful not to quote any.

I cannot imagine your purpose in such a broadcast. It was sickening and misrepresentative throughout. The weakest part was the beginning. Why did the man leave his native land in the first place—to look for a free ride?

Completely disgusted with TV,